SMOKING CONCERNS
SOURCEBOOK

THIRD EDITION

Health Reference Series

SMOKING CONCERNS
SOURCEBOOK

THIRD EDITION

Basic Consumer Health Information about Nicotine Addiction and Smoking Cessation, featuring Facts about the Health Effects of Tobacco Use, including Lung and Other Cancers, Heart Disease, Stroke, and Respiratory Disorders such as Asthma and Chronic Obstructive Pulmonary Disease

Along with Information about Smoking Prevention Programs, Suggestions for Achieving and Maintaining a Smoke-Free Lifestyle, Statistics on Tobacco Use, a Glossary of Terms Related to Smoking, and Directories of Resources for Additional Help and Information

OMNIGRAPHICS
An imprint of Infobase

Bibliographic Note

Because this page cannot legibly accommodate all the copyright notices, the Bibliographic Note portion of the Preface constitutes an extension of the copyright notice.

* * *

OMNIGRAPHICS
An imprint of Infobase
8 The Green
Suite #19225
Dover, DE 19901
www.infobase.com
James Chambers, *Editorial Director*

* * *

ISBN 978-0-7808-2144-6
E-ISBN 978-0-7808-2145-3

Library of Congress Cataloging-in-Publication Data

Names: Chambers, James (Editor), editor. | Omnigraphics, Inc., issuing body.

Title: Smoking concerns sourcebook / edited by James Chambers.

Description: Third edition. | Dover, DE: Omnigraphics, an imprint of Infobase, [2024] | Series: Health reference series | Preceded by: Smoking concerns sourcebook / Angela Williams, managing editor. Second edition. [2019]. | Includes bibliographical references and index. | Summary: "Provides basic consumer health information about nicotine addiction and smoking cessation, with facts about the health effects of tobacco use, including lung and other cancers, heart disease, stroke, as well as respiratory disorders such as asthma and chronic obstructive pulmonary disease. Includes an index, glossary of related terms, and other resources"-- Provided by publisher.

Identifiers: LCCN 2024015145 (print) | LCCN 2024015146 (ebook) | ISBN 9780780821446 (library binding) | ISBN 9780780821453 (ebook)

Subjects: LCSH: Smoking--Health aspects. | Smoking cessation. | Nicotine--Physiological effect.

Classification: LCC RA1242.T6 S589 2024 (print) | LCC RA1242.T6 (ebook) | DDC 613.85--dc23/eng/20240405

LC record available at https://lccn.loc.gov/2024015145

LC ebook record available at https://lccn.loc.gov/2024015146

Printed in the United States

Table of Contents

Part 2. Smoking and Tobacco-Related Health Hazards

Part 3. Smoking Cessation Strategies

Part 4. Tobacco Prevention and Control

Part 5. Additional Help and Information

Preface

ABOUT THIS BOOK

According to the Centers for Disease Control and Prevention (CDC), cigarette smoking remains the leading cause of preventable death in the United States, responsible for over 480,000 deaths annually. This includes more than 41,000 deaths attributed to secondhand smoke exposure. Smoking causes more deaths each year than HIV, illegal drug use, alcohol use, motor vehicle injuries, and firearm-related incidents combined. The financial burden of these illnesses costs the United States over $600 billion annually. Smoking harms nearly every organ in the body and can lead to fatal conditions such as heart disease, cancer, and stroke. Despite the well-documented health risks, quitting smoking remains a significant challenge. Studies indicate that most smokers attempt to quit multiple times before successfully achieving their cessation goals.

Smoking Concerns Sourcebook, Third Edition provides essential information about smoking and tobacco use, offering insights into the effects of nicotine on the body and the development of addiction. The book addresses various aspects of smoking behavior, including gender differences in smoking habits, specific health risks associated with tobacco use, and the challenges of overcoming nicotine dependence. Additionally, it covers methods for managing exposure to secondhand smoke and strategies for maintaining a smoke-free lifestyle. The book concludes with a glossary of terms related to tobacco use and smoking cessation, a directory of resources for further information on tobacco control, and a list of hotlines, helplines, and online resources for those seeking support in their efforts to quit smoking.

HOW TO USE THIS BOOK

This book is divided into parts and chapters. Parts focus on broad areas of interest. Chapters are devoted to single topics within a part.

Part 1: Smoking and Tobacco Use Overview offers an introduction to the harmful substances in tobacco and their effects. It discusses various smoked tobacco products, including cigarettes, cigars, and hookahs, along with emerging products like e-cigarettes and heated tobacco products. The part also addresses gender differences in tobacco use, the effect of cigarette marketing on youth, and the dangers of secondhand and thirdhand smoke.

Part 2: Smoking and Tobacco-Related Health Hazards explores the wide range of health issues linked to smoking, such as increased risks for various cancers, respiratory and cardiovascular diseases, and mental health disorders. It also examines the effects of smoking on specific conditions such as eye disease, Buerger disease, diabetes, and the potential effect of smoking on COVID-19 outcomes.

Part 3: Smoking Cessation Strategies provides detailed guidance on quitting smoking, including creating a personalized quit plan, utilizing nicotine replacement therapy (NRT), and managing withdrawal symptoms. It emphasizes the importance of social support and lifestyle changes post-cessation, while also addressing the unique challenges faced by specific groups, such as women and users of smokeless tobacco.

Part 4: Tobacco Prevention and Control discusses strategies to prevent tobacco use, such as implementing smoke-free policies and promoting smoke-free environments. It also examines the role of media and public policies in shaping tobacco control efforts, the effectiveness of price policies and taxation, and the challenges of reducing tobacco industry influence in the retail environment.

Part 5: Additional Help and Information includes a glossary of terms related to tobacco use and smoking cessation, a directory of resources for further information on tobacco-related issues, and a list of hotlines, helplines, and online resources for smoking cessation support.

BIBLIOGRAPHIC NOTE

This volume contains documents and excerpts from publications issued by the following U.S. government agencies: Centers for Disease Control and Prevention (CDC); Division of Cancer Control and Population Sciences (DCCPS); HIV.gov; National Cancer Institute (NCI); National Heart, Lung, and Blood Institute (NHLBI); National Institute of Dental and Craniofacial Research (NIDCR); National Institute of Diabetes and Digestive and Kidney Diseases (NIDDK); National Institute on Aging (NIA); National Institute on Drug Abuse (NIDA); National Institutes of Health (NIH); Office of Disease Prevention and Health Promotion (ODPHP); Smokefree Teen; Smokefree

Veterans; Smokefree Women; Smokefree.gov; Substance Abuse and Mental Health Services Administration (SAMHSA); U.S. Department of Health and Human Services (HHS); U.S. Department of Veterans Affairs (VA); and U.S. Food and Drug Administration (FDA).

ABOUT THE *HEALTH REFERENCE SERIES*

The *Health Reference Series* is designed to provide basic medical information for patients, families, caregivers, and the general public. Each volume provides comprehensive coverage on a particular topic. This is especially important for people who may be dealing with a newly diagnosed disease or a chronic disorder in themselves or in a family member. People looking for preventive guidance, information about disease warning signs, medical statistics, and risk factors for health problems will also find answers to their questions in the *Health Reference Series*. The *Series*, however, is not intended to serve as a tool for diagnosing illness, in prescribing treatments, or as a substitute for the physician-patient relationship. All people concerned about medical symptoms or the possibility of disease are encouraged to seek professional care from an appropriate health-care provider.

A NOTE ABOUT SPELLING AND STYLE

Health Reference Series editors use *Stedman's Medical Dictionary* as an authority for questions related to the spelling of medical terms and *The Chicago Manual of Style* for questions related to grammatical structures, punctuation, and other editorial concerns. Consistent adherence is not always possible, however, because the individual volumes within the *Series* include many documents from a wide variety of different producers, and the editor's primary goal is to present material from each source as accurately as is possible. This sometimes means that information in different chapters or sections may follow other guidelines and alternate spelling authorities. For example, occasionally a copyright holder may require that eponymous terms be shown in possessive forms (Crohn's disease vs. Crohn disease) or that British spelling norms be retained (leukaemia vs. leukemia).

HEALTH REFERENCE SERIES UPDATE POLICY

The inaugural book in the *Health Reference Series* was the first edition of *Cancer Sourcebook* published in 1989. Since then, the *Series* has been enthusiastically received by librarians and in the medical community. In order to maintain the standard of providing high-quality health information for the layperson, the editorial staff felt it was necessary to implement a policy of updating volumes when warranted.

Medical researchers have been making tremendous strides, and it is the purpose of the *Health Reference Series* to stay current with the most recent advances. Each decision to update a volume is made on an individual basis. Some of the considerations include how much new information is available and the feedback we receive from people who use the books. If there is a topic you would like to see added to the update list, or an area of medical concern you feel has not been adequately addressed, please write to: custserv@infobaselearning.com.

Part 1 | Smoking and Tobacco Use Overview

Chapter 1 | **Understanding the Effects of Tobacco Smoking**

OVERVIEW

Smoking leads to disease and disability and harms nearly every organ of the body. It remains the leading cause of preventable disease, disability, and death in the United States. The tobacco industry spends billions of dollars each year on marketing cigarettes, while smoking costs the United States hundreds of billions of dollars annually.[1]

- On average, compared to people who have never smoked:
  - smokers suffer for years with more health problems due to their smoking
  - smokers ultimately die earlier by a decade or more than nonsmokers
- Smokers generally are much less healthy than nonsmokers, experiencing:
  - worse overall health
  - more frequent illness
  - increased doctor visits
  - higher hospital admission rates
- Additionally, smokers miss more work than nonsmokers, costing:
  - American businesses billions of dollars every year
  - American workers who smoke billions of dollars every year[2]

[1] "Fast Facts and Fact Sheets," Centers for Disease Control and Prevention (CDC), November 2, 2023. Available online. URL: www.cdc.gov/tobacco/data_statistics/fact_sheets/fast_facts/index.htm. Accessed March 27, 2024.
[2] "Smoking and Overall Health," Centers for Disease Control and Prevention (CDC), May 28, 2016. Available online. URL: www.cdc.gov/tobacco/data_statistics/sgr/50th-anniversary/pdfs/fs_smoking_overall_health_508.pdf. Accessed March 21, 2024.

REASONS FOR SMOKING

People use tobacco for various reasons, including stress relief, pleasure, or social situations.

Addiction

Nicotine, the main addictive substance in cigarettes and other forms of tobacco, affects many parts of the body, including the brain. Over time, the body and brain get used to having nicotine, leading to addiction in about 80–90 percent of regular smokers.

Nicotine reaches the brain within 10 seconds of entering the body, causing the release of adrenaline and creating a buzz of pleasure and energy. This buzz quickly fades, leaving the smoker feeling tired or down, and wanting that buzz again. The body builds up a high tolerance to nicotine, requiring more cigarettes to achieve the same buzz, leading to a cycle of addiction.

When people do not smoke, they may experience withdrawal symptoms as their bodies adjust to the absence of nicotine. Withdrawal symptoms may include:

- feeling down or sad
- trouble sleeping
- irritability, on edge, grouchy
- difficulty thinking clearly and concentrating
- restlessness and jumpiness
- slower heart rate
- increased hunger or weight gain

Nicotine replacement therapy (NRT) can help reduce cravings and withdrawal symptoms. Your health-care providers can prescribe NRT, which is also available over the counter at local pharmacies.

Patterns

Smoking often becomes connected to daily activities, such as watching TV, talking on the phone, hanging out with friends, visiting certain places, or taking a break to relax. This connection creates a pattern or routine.

Help is available to break this routine. In-person counseling or telephone counseling can teach you how to dissociate smoking from daily activities and create new, healthier patterns.

Emotions

Many people smoke to cope with posttraumatic stress disorder (PTSD) symptoms, negative moods, and daily stress. However, there are healthier ways to deal with emotions. Counseling can teach you coping strategies, and support from loved ones can also help.

Understanding the reasons behind smoking and recognizing its severe effects on health are crucial steps toward quitting. With proper support and resources, such as nicotine replacement therapy, counseling, and emotional support, smokers can break free from addiction and develop healthier habits.[3]

[3] Smokefree Veterans, "Reasons People Smoke," U.S. Department of Health and Human Services (HHS), February 24, 2017. Available online. URL: https://veterans.smokefree.gov/nicotine-addiction/reasons-people-smoke. Accessed March 21, 2024.

Chapter 2 | **Understanding the Dangers of Tobacco Use**

OVERVIEW

A plant with leaves that have high levels of the addictive chemical nicotine, tobacco is processed into various products after harvesting, curing, aging, and processing. These products may be smoked (in cigarettes, cigars, and pipes), applied to the gums (as dipping and chewing tobacco), or inhaled (as snuff). Cured tobacco leaves and the products made from them contain many cancer-causing chemicals, and tobacco use and exposure to secondhand tobacco smoke have been strongly linked to many types of cancer and other diseases.[1]

REGULATORY MEASURES AND REPORTING

The FDA and FD&C Act

The Food, Drug, and Cosmetic Act (FD&C Act) requires tobacco manufacturers and importers to report the levels of harmful and potentially harmful constituents (HPHCs) found in their tobacco products and tobacco smoke. HPHCs are chemicals in tobacco products or smoke that cause or could cause harm to smokers or nonsmokers.

The U.S. Food and Drug Administration (FDA) must publish HPHC quantities in each brand and subbrand of tobacco product in a way that is understandable and not misleading. Several efforts are underway at the FDA to progress toward this goal.

[1] "Tobacco," National Cancer Institute (NCI), March 31, 2017. Available online. URL: www.cancer.gov/publications/dictionaries/cancer-terms/def/tobacco. Accessed April 8, 2024.

Preliminary HPHC List

In March 2012, the FDA published a preliminary list of 93 HPHCs, focusing on chemicals linked to the most serious health effects of tobacco use (cancer, cardiovascular disease (CVD), respiratory effects, reproductive problems, and addiction).

The list of HPHCs in tobacco products and tobacco smoke as required by the FD&C Act is included in Table 2.1.

Table 2.1. Established List of the Chemicals and Chemical Compounds

Constituent	Carcinogen (CA), Respiratory Toxicant (RT), Cardiovascular Toxicant (CT), Reproductive or Developmental Toxicant (RDT), Addictive (AD)
Acetaldehyde	CA, RT, AD
Acetamide	CA
Acetone	RT
Acrolein	RT, CT
Acrylamide	CA
Acrylonitrile	CA, RT
Aflatoxin B1	CA
4-Aminobiphenyl	CA
1-Aminonaphthalene	CA
2-Aminonaphthalene	CA
Ammonia	RT
Anabasine	AD
o-Anisidine	CA
Arsenic	CA, CT, RDT
A-α-C (2-Amino-9H-pyrido[2,3-b]indole)	CA
Benz[a]anthracene	CA, CT
Benz[j]aceanthrylene	CA

Table 2.1. Continued

Constituent	Carcinogen (CA), Respiratory Toxicant (RT), Cardiovascular Toxicant (CT), Reproductive or Developmental Toxicant (RDT), Addictive (AD)
Benzene	CA, CT, RDT
Benzo[b]fluoranthene	CA, CT
Benzo[k]fluoranthene	CA, CT
Benzo[b]furan	CA
Benzo[a]pyrene	CA
Benzo[c]phenanthrene	CA
Beryllium	CA
1,3-Butadiene	CA, RT, RDT
Cadmium	CA, RT, RDT
Caffeic acid	CA
Carbon monoxide	RDT
Catechol	CA
Chlorinated dioxins/furans	CA, RDT
Chromium	CA, RT, RDT
Chrysene	CA, CT
Cobalt	CA, CT
Coumarin	Banned in food
Cresols (o-, m-, and p-cresol)	CA, RT
Crotonaldehyde	CA
Cyclopenta[c,d]pyrene	CA
Dibenz[a,h]anthracene	CA
Dibenzo[a,e]pyrene	CA
Dibenzo[a,h]pyrene	CA

Table 2.1. Continued

Constituent	**Carcinogen (CA), Respiratory Toxicant (RT), Cardiovascular Toxicant (CT), Reproductive or Developmental Toxicant (RDT), Addictive (AD)**
Dibenzo[a,i]pyrene	CA
Dibenzo[a,l]pyrene	CA
2,6-Dimethylaniline	CA
Ethyl carbamate (urethane)	CA, RDT
Ethylbenzene	CA
Ethylene oxide	CA, RT, RDT
Formaldehyde	CA, RT
Furan	CA
Glu-P-1 (2-Amino-6-methyldipyrido[1,2-a:3',2'-d] imidazole)	CA
Glu-P-2 (2-Aminodipyrido[1,2-a:3',2'-d]imidazole)	CA
Hydrazine	CA, RT
Hydrogen cyanide	RT, CT
Indeno[1,2,3-cd]pyrene	CA
IQ (2-Amino-3-methylimidazo[4,5-f]quinoline)	CA
Isoprene	CA
Lead	CA, CT, RDT
MeA-α-C (2-Amino-3-methyl)-9H-pyrido[2,3-b] indole)	CA
Mercury	CA, RDT
Methyl ethyl ketone	RT
5-Methylchrysene	CA
4-(Methylnitrosamino)-1-(3-pyridyl)-1-butanone (NNK)	CA

Table 2.1. Continued

Constituent	**Carcinogen (CA), Respiratory Toxicant (RT), Cardiovascular Toxicant (CT), Reproductive or Developmental Toxicant (RDT), Addictive (AD)**
Naphthalene	CA, RT
Nickel	CA, RT
Nicotine	RDT, AD
Nitrobenzene	CA, RT, RDT
Nitromethane	CA
2-Nitropropane	CA
N-Nitrosodiethanolamine (NDELA)	CA
N-Nitrosodiethylamine	CA
N-Nitrosodimethylamine (NDMA)	CA
N-Nitrosomethylethylamine	CA
N-Nitrosomorpholine (NMOR)	CA
N-Nitrosonornicotine (NNN)	CA
N-Nitrosopiperidine (NPIP)	CA
N-Nitrosopyrrolidine (NPYR)	CA
N-Nitrososarcosine (NSAR)	CA
Nornicotine	AD
Phenol	RT, CT
PhIP (2-Amino-1-methyl-6-phenylimidazo[4,5-b] pyridine)	CA
Polonium-210	CA
Propionaldehyde	RT, CT
Propylene oxide	CA, RT
Quinoline	CA

Table 2.1. Continued

Constituent	Carcinogen (CA), Respiratory Toxicant (RT), Cardiovascular Toxicant (CT), Reproductive or Developmental Toxicant (RDT), Addictive (AD)
Selenium	RT
Styrene	CA
o-Toluidine	CA
Toluene	RT, RDT
Trp-P-1 (3-Amino-1,4-dimethyl-5H-pyrido[4,3-b] indole)	CA
Trp-P-2 (1-Methyl-3-amino-5H-pyrido[4,3-b] indole)	CA
Uranium-235	CA, RT
Uranium-238	CA, RT
Vinyl acetate	CA, RT
Vinyl chloride	CA

Tobacco Industry Reporting Requirements

The FDA issued draft guidance in 2012 that identified a subset of 20 HPHCs for which manufacturers and importers must test and report to the FDA. These 20 HPHCs were chosen because testing methods were well established and widely available. The FDA is now evaluating the quality and reliability of the data submitted by manufacturers.

COMMUNICATING RISKS TO THE PUBLIC

The FDA is researching how best to ensure the public is aware of the dangers of chemicals and compounds in tobacco products and smoke and to communicate the levels of HPHCs in each brand and subbrand of tobacco product.[2]

[2] "Harmful and Potentially Harmful Constituents (HPHCs)," U.S. Food and Drug Administration (FDA), October 7, 2019. Available online. URL: www.fda.gov/tobacco-products/products-ingredients-components/harmful-and-potentially-harmful-constituents-hphcs. Accessed April 8, 2024.

CIGARETTE SMOKING AND RADIATION

Cigarette smoke and tobacco contain many toxic substances, including tar, arsenic, nicotine, and cyanide. However, few people know that tobacco also contains radioactive materials, such as polonium-210 and lead-210. These materials accumulate in the lungs of smokers and can lead to lung cancer. The Centers for Disease Control and Prevention (CDC) estimates that smoking causes 80 percent of all lung cancer deaths in women and 90 percent of all lung cancer deaths in men.[3]

HOW TOBACCO DELIVERS ITS EFFECTS

The smoke from combustible tobacco products contains more than 7,000 chemicals. Nicotine is the primary reinforcing component of tobacco, driving addiction. Hundreds of compounds are added to tobacco to enhance its flavor and the absorption of nicotine. Cigarette smoking is the most popular method of using tobacco, but many people also use smokeless tobacco products, such as snuff and chewing tobacco, which also contain nicotine.

By inhaling tobacco smoke, the average smoker takes in 1–2 milligrams of nicotine per cigarette. Nicotine rapidly reaches peak levels in the bloodstream and enters the brain, causing a "kick" by stimulating the adrenal glands and releasing adrenaline. This rush increases blood pressure, respiration, and heart rate, and activates reward pathways in the brain, reinforcing feelings of pleasure.[4]

PREVENTING AND HELPING PEOPLE QUIT TOBACCO PRODUCTS

Actions for Parents and Teachers

- Learn about menthol and its relationship to tobacco product use and nicotine dependence among young people.
- Take advantage of quitting resources in their community if they use tobacco products.

---

[3] "Facts about Cigarette Smoking and Radiation," Centers for Disease Control and Prevention (CDC), February 20, 2024. Available online. URL: www.cdc.gov/radiation-health/data-research/facts-stats/cigarette-smoking.html. Accessed July 22, 2024.

[4] "How Does Tobacco Deliver Its Effects?" National Institute on Drug Abuse (NIDA), March 25, 2021. Available online. URL: https://nida.nih.gov/publications/research-reports/tobacco-nicotine-e-cigarettes/how-does-tobacco-deliver-its-effects. Accessed April 8, 2024.

- Talk to children, teens, and young adults about the harms of all forms of tobacco products.
- Develop and enforce tobacco-free school policies that address all types of tobacco products and incorporate nonpunitive penalties.
- Implement school prevention and cessation programs that are free from tobacco industry influence and can be tailored to targeted groups.

Actions for Health Professionals

- Learn about menthol and its relationship to tobacco use, nicotine dependence, and reduced cessation success.
- Learn about different types of tobacco products and their risks.
- Screen all patients for tobacco product use.
- Encourage patients to quit using tobacco products and provide information about evidence-based quitting resources, including counseling and medication.[5]

[5] "Addressing Menthol Tobacco Products," Centers for Disease Control and Prevention (CDC), May 15, 2024. Available online. URL: www.cdc.gov/tobacco/menthol-tobacco/addressing-products.html. Accessed April 9, 2024.

Chapter 3 | Smoked Tobacco Products

Chapter Contents

Section 3.1 | **Cigarettes**

WHAT ARE CIGARETTES?

Cigarettes are still the most commonly used tobacco product in the United States. They are also responsible for the vast majority of all tobacco-related diseases and deaths in the country.

COMPONENTS AND HARMFUL EFFECTS

The basic components of most cigarettes are:

- tobacco
- chemical additives
- a filter
- paper wrapping

When the tobacco is burned, the smoke is inhaled. People who smoke are exposed to a toxic mix of over 7,000 chemicals, including more than 70 that can cause cancer.[1]

STATISTICS OF CIGARETTE SMOKING IN THE UNITED STATES

Prevalence of Smoking among Adults (2021)

- Overall: 11.5 percent of all adults (28.3 million people)
    - Men: 13.1 percent
    - Women: 10.1 percent
- By Race/Ethnicity:
    - Non-Hispanic adults from other racial groups: 14.9 percent
    - Non-Hispanic white adults: 12.9 percent
    - Non-Hispanic Black adults: 11.7 percent
    - Hispanic adults: 7.7 percent
    - Non-Hispanic Asian adults: 5.4 percent

[1] "Cigarettes," U.S. Food and Drug Administration (FDA), June 7, 2023. Available online. URL: www.fda.gov/tobacco-products/products-ingredients-components/cigarettes. Accessed April 9, 2024.

Note: *Current cigarette smokers are defined as people who reported smoking at least 100 cigarettes during their lifetime and who, at the time they participated in a survey about this topic, reported smoking every day or some days. 2021 tobacco product estimates for American Indian/Alaska Native adults were not statistically reliable.*

Youth Smoking Initiation

- Each day, about 2,000 people younger than 18 years smoke their first cigarette.
- Each day, over 300 people younger than 18 years become daily cigarette smokers.

Efforts and Success in Quitting Smoking

- In 2015, nearly 7 in 10 (68.0%) adult cigarette smokers wanted to stop smoking.
- In 2018, more than half (55.1%) of adult cigarette smokers had made a quit attempt in the past year.
- In 2018, more than 7 out of every 100 (7.5%) people who tried to quit succeeded.
- From 2012 to 2018, the "Tips From Former Smokers" campaign motivated approximately 1 million tobacco smokers to quit for good.

Note: "*Made a quit attempt*" *refers to smokers who reported that they stopped smoking for more than one day in the past 12 months because they were trying to quit smoking.*

Cigarettes remain a significant health risk, contributing to numerous diseases and deaths each year. Efforts to reduce smoking rates and help smokers quit are ongoing and critical to improving public health.[2]

[2] "Cigarette Smoking in the U.S.," Centers for Disease Control and Prevention (CDC), May 4, 2023. Available online. URL: www.cdc.gov/tobacco/data_statistics/fact_sheets/fast_facts/cigarette-smoking-in-the-us.html. Accessed April 9, 2024.

Section 3.2 | **Cigars and Cigarillos**

WHAT ARE CIGARS?

A cigar is defined as a roll of tobacco wrapped in leaf tobacco or in a substance that contains tobacco. Cigars differ from cigarettes in that cigarettes are a roll of tobacco wrapped in paper or in a substance that does not contain tobacco.

The three major types of cigars (see Table 3.1) sold in the United States are:

- large cigars
- cigarillos
- little cigars

Table 3.1. Description and Unit Sale Share of Cigar Types

Type	Description	Share of Unit Sales (2016–2020)*
Large cigar	A cigar that typically contains at least one-half ounce of aged, fermented tobacco (i.e., as much as a pack of cigarettes) and usually takes one to two hours to smoke.	2.70 percent
Cigarillo	A short (3–4 inches) and narrow cigar that typically contains about 3 grams of tobacco and usually does not include a filter.	94.20 percent
Little cigar	A small cigar that typically is about the same size as a cigarette and usually includes a filter.	3.10 percent

* *Percentage of U.S. market for cigar products.*

USAGE AMONG YOUTH

In 2023, cigars were the third most commonly used tobacco product among U.S. middle and high school students. The availability of flavors in cigars that are prohibited in cigarettes (such as cherry) and the fact that they are commonly sold as a single stick has raised concerns that these products may be especially appealing to youth. In 2021, among middle and high school students who used cigars in the past 30 days, 44.4 percent reported using a flavored cigar during that time. Little cigars are the same size and shape as cigarettes, often include a filter, and are packaged similarly, but they are taxed differently. Rather than reduce consumption, people who smoke and are cost-conscious might switch from cigarettes to cheaper little cigars.

HISTORICAL AND CURRENT TRENDS

Historically, cigar smoking in the United States has been a behavior of older men. However, the industry's increased marketing of these products to targeted groups has increased the prevalence of use among adolescents. Cigar use is higher among youth who use other tobacco products or other drugs (e.g., alcohol, marijuana, and inhalants) than among youth who do not use these products.

HEALTH EFFECTS

Cigars, whether they are large cigars, cigarillos, or little cigars, pose significant health risks to users. They contain the same toxic and carcinogenic compounds found in cigarettes and are not a safe alternative. Regularly smoking cigars is associated with an increased risk for:

- cancers of the lung, esophagus, larynx (voice box), and oral cavity (lip, tongue, mouth, throat)
- gum disease and tooth loss
- coronary heart disease, particularly with heavy cigar smoking and deep inhalation of cigar smoke
- lung diseases, such as emphysema and chronic bronchitis

CURRENT CIGAR USE

Adults (2021)

- Overall: 3.5 percent of all adults
  - Men: 6.2 percent
  - Women: 1.0 percent

- Non-Hispanic Black adults: 5.1 percent
- Non-Hispanic white adults: 3.7 percent
- Hispanic adults: 2.5 percent
- Non-Hispanic Asian adults: 1.2 percent

High School Students (2023)

- Overall: 1.8 percent of all students in grades 9–12
  - Female students: 1.4 percent
  - Male students: 2.3 percent

Middle School Students (2023)

- Overall: 1.1 percent of all U.S. students in grades 6–8
  - Female students: 1.2 percent
  - Male students: 1.0 percent

In 2021, an estimated 8.6 million adults aged 18 and older (3.5%) smoked cigars.

Note: *Current cigar use is defined as smoking cigars on one or more of the 30 days before participation in a survey about this topic.*

MARKETING INFORMATION

Marketing efforts promote cigars as symbols of a luxurious and successful lifestyle. The following strategies contribute to the increased acceptability of cigar smoking:

- endorsements by male and female celebrities
- development of cigar-focused magazines (e.g., Cigar Aficionado)
- product placement in movies

Despite their different forms and marketing strategies, cigars are not a safe alternative to cigarettes. The increased marketing of flavored and single-stick cigars raises concerns about their appeal to youth, further complicating public health efforts.

REGULATORY MEASURES

In 2001, the Federal Trade Commission (FTC) mandated that cigar packaging and advertisements display one of the following five "SURGEON GENERAL WARNING" text-only labels on a rotating basis:

1. Cigar Smoking Can Cause Cancers of the Mouth and Throat, Even If You Do Not Inhale.
2. Cigar Smoking Can Cause Lung Cancer and Heart Disease.
3. Tobacco Use Increases the Risk of Infertility, Stillbirth, and Low Birth Weight.
4. Cigars are Not a Safe Alternative to Cigarettes.
5. Tobacco Smoke Increases the Risk of Lung Cancer and Heart Disease, Even in Nonsmokers.

It is crucial to understand the dangers associated with all types of cigars and to take measures to reduce their consumption and mitigate their health effects.[1]

Section 3.3 | **Hookahs**

WHAT IS A HOOKAH?

Hookahs, or *narghile*, *argileh*, *shisha*, hubble-bubble, and *goza*, are water pipes used to smoke specially made tobacco in different flavors such as apple, mint, cherry, chocolate, coconut, licorice, cappuccino, and watermelon. Despite common misconceptions, hookah smoking carries many of the same health risks as cigarette smoking.

HOOKAH COMPONENTS AND USAGE

A typical modern hookah has:

- a head with holes in the bottom
- a metal body

[1] "Cigars," Centers for Disease Control and Prevention (CDC), November 2, 2023. Available online. URL: www.cdc.gov/tobacco/data_statistics/fact_sheets/tobacco_industry/cigars/index.htm. Accessed April 9, 2024.

- a water bowl
- a flexible hose with a mouthpiece

Hookah smoking is typically done in groups, with the same mouthpiece passed from person to person. This practice is not a safe alternative to smoking cigarettes. People who use tobacco should quit all tobacco products to reduce health risks.

HOOKAH USE STATISTICS

- Historical background:
  - Hookah use began centuries ago in ancient Persia and India.
- Recent usage:
  - In 2018, nearly 1 in every 13 (7.8%) high school students in the United States had used a hookah to smoke tobacco in the previous year.
  - About one in every eight (12.3%) young adults aged 19–30 years had used a hookah to smoke tobacco in the previous year.
  - Among 12th graders, annual hookah use increased from nearly 1 in 6 students (17.1%) in 2010 to about 1 in 4 students (22.9%) in 2014, but sharply decreased to nearly 1 in 13 students (7.8%) in 2018.
  - In 2018, the highest prevalence of use was observed in the Northeast (15.0%) and in very large cities (19.3%) among young adults aged 19–30 years.
  - Other studies show past-year use ranging from 22 to 40 percent among U.S. college students.

NEW FORMS OF ELECTRONIC HOOKAH PRODUCTS

New electronic hookah products, such as steam stones and hookah pens, have been introduced. These battery-powered products turn liquid containing nicotine, flavorings, and other chemicals into an aerosol, which is inhaled. Limited information is currently available on the health risks of electronic tobacco products, including electronic hookahs.

HEALTH EFFECTS OF HOOKAH SMOKE

Cancer Risks

- **Toxic agents.** Hookah tobacco and smoke contain several toxic agents known to cause lung, bladder, and oral cancers.
- **Charcoal use.** The charcoal used to heat the tobacco can produce high levels of carbon monoxide, metals, and cancer-causing chemicals.
- **Oral cancers.** Tobacco juices from hookahs irritate the mouth and increase the risk of developing oral cancers.

Other Health Risks

- **Cardiovascular disease (CVD).** Hookah tobacco and smoke contain many toxic agents that can cause clogged arteries and heart disease.
- **Pregnancy risks.** Babies born to people who smoke water pipes every day while pregnant weigh less at birth and are at increased risk for respiratory diseases.

COMPARING HOOKAH AND CIGARETTE SMOKING

- **Harmful components.** Hookah smoke contains many of the same harmful components found in cigarette smoke, such as nicotine, tar, and heavy metals.
- **Nicotine delivery.** Water pipe smoking delivers nicotine, the same highly addictive drug found in other tobacco products.
- **Heat source risks.** The heat sources used to burn hookah tobacco release dangerous substances like carbon monoxide.
- **Smoke inhalation.** In a typical one-hour hookah smoking session, users may inhale 100–200 times the amount of smoke they would from a single cigarette.
- **Exposure.** Users are exposed to up to 9 times the carbon monoxide and 1.7 times the nicotine of a single cigarette.

- **Health risks**. Hookah smokers may be at risk for the same diseases as cigarette smokers, including oral, lung, stomach, and esophagus cancers, reduced lung function, and decreased fertility.

HOOKAHS AND SECONDHAND SMOKE

Secondhand smoke from hookahs contains smoke from both the tobacco and the heat source (e.g., charcoal), posing health risks to nonsmokers.

NONTOBACCO HOOKAH PRODUCTS

Some sweetened and flavored nontobacco products are sold for use in hookahs. Despite claims that these products are safer, studies show that smoke from both tobacco-based and "herbal" shisha contains carbon monoxide and other toxic agents that increase risks for smoking-related cancers, heart disease, and lung disease.[1]

[1] "Hookahs," Centers for Disease Control and Prevention (CDC), April 22, 2021. Available online. URL: www.cdc.gov/tobacco/data_statistics/fact_sheets/tobacco_industry/hookahs/index.htm. Accessed April 9, 2024.

Chapter 4 | **Cigarette Variants**

Chapter Contents

Section 4.1 | Light Cigarettes

Since the 1950s, tobacco manufacturers have redesigned cigarettes with features marketed as "light" cigarettes. These features include cellulose acetate filters, highly porous cigarette paper, ventilation holes in the filter tip, and different blends of tobacco. While these design changes lower tar yields when analyzed by smoking machines, studies show they do not reduce the risk of disease caused by smoking.

THE FAMILY SMOKING PREVENTION AND TOBACCO CONTROL ACT

On June 22, 2009, President Barack Obama signed the Family Smoking Prevention and Tobacco Control Act, granting the U.S. Food and Drug Administration (FDA) authority to regulate tobacco products. This law bans the use of the terms "light," "low," and "mild" in product labeling and advertisements, effective June 22, 2010. However, some manufacturers continue to market these products misleadingly using color-coded packaging.

HEALTH RISKS OF LIGHT CIGARETTES

Are Light Cigarettes Less Hazardous than Regular Cigarettes?

No. Light cigarettes are no safer than regular cigarettes. Tar exposure from a light cigarette can be as high as from a regular cigarette, depending on how the smoker puffs. The only way to reduce health risks from smoking is to quit entirely.

Do Light Cigarettes Cause Cancer?

Yes. Smoking any kind of cigarette greatly increases the risk of lung cancer and other diseases. Smokers of light cigarettes inhale similar amounts of toxic chemicals as those who smoke regular cigarettes, maintaining a high risk of developing smoking-related cancers and other diseases. Smoking causes cancers of the lung, esophagus, larynx, mouth, throat, kidney, bladder, pancreas, stomach, and cervix, as well as acute myeloid leukemia (AML). Quitting smoking reduces these risks substantially.

MISLEADING TAR YIELD RATINGS

Tar Yield Ratings for Light Cigarettes

The tobacco industry used specific tar yield ranges to categorize cigarettes:

- **Ultralight or Ultralow tar.** Usually 7 milligrams or less.
- **Light or Low tar.** Usually 8–14 milligrams.
- **Full flavor or Regular.** Usually 15 milligrams or more.

These ratings were not accurate indicators of actual tar exposure, as smokers do not smoke cigarettes the same way machines do.

Are Machine-Measured Tar Yields Misleading?

Yes. Machine-measured tar yields cannot predict actual tar intake because smokers often take deeper, longer, and more frequent puffs than the machine. This can lead to greater tar exposure, with smokers potentially blocking air ventilation holes in the filter.[1]

COMPENSATORY SMOKING BEHAVIOR

People addicted to nicotine may compensate by taking bigger puffs, inhaling more deeply, or smoking more cigarettes to satisfy their cravings. This leads to a higher intake of tar, nicotine, and other harmful chemicals, negating the intended benefits of light cigarettes. Tobacco industry documents reveal that companies were aware of this compensatory behavior and the difference between machine-measured yields and actual smoker inhalation.[2]

QUITTING SMOKING

Quitting smoking is the best way to reduce the health risks associated with tobacco use. There are many resources available to help smokers quit, including:

- **Smokefree.gov (www.smokefree.gov).** Offers a step-by-step quit guide.

---

[1] "'Light' Cigarettes and Cancer Risk," National Cancer Institute (NCI), October 28, 2010. Available online. URL: www.cancer.gov/about-cancer/causes-prevention/risk/tobacco/light-cigarettes-fact-sheet. Accessed April 8, 2024.

[2] "Low-Yield Cigarettes," Centers for Disease Control and Prevention (CDC), March 25, 2021. Available online. URL: www.cdc.gov/tobacco/data_statistics/fact_sheets/tobacco_industry/low_yield_cigarettes/index.htm. Accessed April 8, 2024.

- **National Cancer Institute's (NCI) smoking quitline.** Call 1-877-44U-QUIT (1-877-448-7848) for individualized counseling and referrals.
- **NCI fact sheet.** Where To Get Help When You Decide To Quit Smoking (www.cancer.gov/about-cancer/causes-prevention/risk/tobacco/help-quitting-fact-sheet).

Light cigarettes are not a safer alternative to regular cigarettes. Both types contain harmful chemicals that pose significant health risks. The only way to effectively reduce these risks is to quit smoking entirely.[3]

Section 4.2 | Menthol Cigarettes

Menthol is a chemical added to cigarettes and other tobacco products, making them more addictive than regular cigarettes. It has been marketed to young people and other groups to encourage them to start and keep smoking.

WHAT IS MENTHOL?

Menthol is a chemical naturally found in peppermint and other plants and can also be made in a lab. It is one of the most commonly used flavorings in tobacco products. Tobacco companies add menthol to cigarettes and other tobacco products to make them more appealing and to encourage people to keep smoking.

Menthol masks the harsh taste and irritation of cigarette smoke, making it easier for people, especially young people, to begin and continue using cigarettes. This results in people who smoke menthol cigarettes tending to smoke more and inhale more deeply than those who smoke nonmenthol cigarettes.

[3] See footnote [1].

Some people believe that menthol cigarettes are safer than nonmenthol cigarettes, but this is not true. Like nonmenthol cigarettes, menthol cigarettes harm nearly every organ in the body and cause many diseases, such as cancer and heart disease. Quitting is the best thing you can do for your health if you smoke menthol cigarettes.

WHO USES MENTHOL CIGARETTES?

Young people, Black/African-American people, other racial and ethnic groups, women, people with lower incomes, people with mental health conditions, and people who identify as LGBTQ+ are more likely to use menthol cigarettes than other groups. For many decades, tobacco companies have targeted certain groups with menthol cigarette marketing. This targeted marketing is a major reason for tobacco-related health disparities in some groups.

Menthol cigarettes contain nicotine, the main addictive drug in tobacco products. Menthol enhances the effect of nicotine on the brain, making menthol cigarettes even more addictive than nonmenthol cigarettes. Even though fewer people are smoking now than in the past, the percentage of people who smoke menthol cigarettes has declined more slowly than the percentage of people who smoke nonmenthol cigarettes.

Menthol cigarettes, including how and to whom they are marketed and sold, pose a significant risk to public health and advancing health equity due to their role in initiation, progression to regular smoking and dependence, reduced cessation success, and contribution to health disparities.[1]

TOBACCO INDUSTRY'S TARGETED MARKETING OF MENTHOL PRODUCTS

The tobacco industry targets menthol cigarette marketing to certain populations through advertisements, giveaways, lower prices, lifestyle branding, and event sponsorships. For example, tobacco companies have heavily marketed in Black-owned publications,

[1] Smokefree.gov, "Quitting Menthol Tobacco," U.S. Department of Health and Human Services (HHS), November 23, 2023. Available online. URL: https://smokefree.gov/quit-smoking/ecigs-menthol-dip/quitting-menthol-tobacco. Accessed April 9, 2024.

through sponsorship of jazz concerts and certain civil rights groups, through advertisements showing people dressed in clothing popular with rap and hip-hop artists, and in neighborhoods with more Black residents. These aggressive marketing tactics have likely contributed to some groups having higher rates of use than others. Given how menthol interacts with nicotine, people who smoke menthol cigarettes are more likely to continue smoking, putting them at higher risk of tobacco-related diseases.

The tobacco industry uses similar strategies to market menthol cigars. For example, tobacco companies have published advertisements in newspapers with a large proportion of Black readers. More recently, the industry has advertised menthol cigars on social media and used hip-hop and rap artists, models, and music appealing to youth.

No tobacco product is safe, including those with menthol. Despite this, tobacco companies market menthol cigarettes as smoother than other cigarettes, and marketing messages imply that menthol cigarettes are a healthier alternative.

EFFECTS OF MENTHOL ON INITIATION AND DEPENDENCE IN YOUTH AND YOUNG ADULTS

Menthol makes cigarettes more appealing and easier to smoke. In addition, menthol enhances the addictive effects of nicotine in the brain. The amount of nicotine in menthol cigarettes has increased in recent years.

Menthol in cigarettes makes it more likely that youth and young adults will try smoking and that those who start smoking will continue on a regular basis.

Tobacco companies have conducted extensive research on menthol. They adjust the amount of menthol in cigarette brands to make each brand most appealing to the people they target. For example, the companies lowered the amount of menthol in some brands to make them more appealing to young people who smoke and those just starting to smoke. They increased the amount of menthol in other brands to make them more appealing to older people.

Menthol in other tobacco products can also lead to continued use. For example, youth and young adults whose first cigar was flavored with mint or menthol were 72 percent more likely to use cigars a year or more later than those whose first cigar was not flavored.

MENTHOL'S EFFECT ON SMOKING CESSATION EFFORTS

People who smoke menthol cigarettes are less likely to successfully quit than those who smoke nonmenthol cigarettes. For example, young adults and adults who smoke menthol cigarettes make more attempts to quit smoking than those who smoke nonmenthol cigarettes. However, the proportion of people who tried and succeeded in quitting nonmenthol cigarettes is greater than the proportion who have tried and succeeded in quitting menthol cigarettes. This could be partly due to how menthol enhances the addictive effects of nicotine in the brain.[2]

Section 4.3 | E-cigarettes (Vapes)

Electronic cigarettes (e-cigarettes) have the potential to benefit adults who smoke and are not pregnant if used as a complete substitute for regular cigarettes and other smoked tobacco products. E-cigarettes, however, are not safe for youth, young adults, pregnant adults, and adults who do not currently use tobacco products. While e-cigarettes may benefit some people and harm others, scientists still have much to learn about whether e-cigarettes are effective in helping adults quit smoking. If you have never smoked or used other tobacco products or e-cigarettes, do not start.

WHAT ARE E-CIGARETTES?

E-cigarettes are sometimes called "e-cigs," "vapes," "e-hookahs," "vape pens," and "electronic nicotine delivery systems" (ENDS).

[2] "Menthol Tobacco Products Are a Public Health Problem," Centers for Disease Control and Prevention (CDC), May 15, 2024. Available online. URL: www.cdc.gov/tobacco/menthol-tobacco/public-health-problem.html. Accessed July 22, 2024.

Some look like regular cigarettes, cigars, or pipes, while others resemble USB flash drives, pens, and other everyday items.

E-cigarettes come in many shapes and sizes, most containing a battery, a heating element, and a place to hold a liquid. E-cigarettes produce an aerosol by heating a liquid that usually contains nicotine—the addictive drug in regular cigarettes, cigars, and other tobacco products—flavorings, and other chemicals that help create the aerosol. Users inhale this aerosol into their lungs. Bystanders can also breathe in this aerosol when the user exhales into the air. Larger devices, such as tank systems or mods, do not resemble other tobacco products. Using an e-cigarette is sometimes called "vaping." E-cigarettes can also be used to deliver marijuana and other drugs.

WHAT IS IN E-CIGARETTE AEROSOL?

The e-cigarette aerosol that users breathe from the device and exhale can contain harmful and potentially harmful substances, including:

- nicotine
- ultrafine particles that can be inhaled deep into the lungs
- flavorings such as diacetyl, a chemical linked to serious lung disease
- volatile organic compounds
- cancer-causing chemicals
- heavy metals such as nickel, tin, and lead

It is difficult for consumers to know what e-cigarette products contain. For example, some e-cigarettes marketed as containing 0 percent nicotine have been found to contain nicotine.

HEALTH EFFECTS OF USING E-CIGARETTES

E-cigarettes are still fairly new, and scientists are still learning about their long-term health effects.

Most e-cigarettes contain nicotine, which has known health effects:

- nicotine is highly addictive
- nicotine is toxic to developing fetuses

- nicotine can harm adolescent and young adult brain development, which continues into the early to mid-20s
- nicotine is a health danger for pregnant adults and their developing babies

Besides nicotine, e-cigarette aerosol can contain substances that harm the body, including cancer-causing chemicals and tiny particles that reach deep into the lungs. However, e-cigarette aerosol generally contains fewer harmful chemicals than smoke from burned tobacco products.

E-cigarettes can cause unintended injuries. Defective e-cigarette batteries have caused fires and explosions, some of which have resulted in serious injuries. Most explosions happened when the e-cigarette batteries were being charged. The Food and Drug Administration (FDA) collects data to help address this issue. You can report an e-cigarette explosion or any unexpected health or safety issue with an e-cigarette at www.fda.gov/tobacco-products/tobacco-science-research/safety-reporting-portal-tobacco-products.

In addition, acute nicotine exposure can be toxic. Children and adults have been poisoned by swallowing, breathing, or absorbing e-cigarette liquid through their skin or eyes.

RISKS OF E-CIGARETTES FOR YOUTH, YOUNG ADULTS, AND PREGNANT ADULTS

Most e-cigarettes contain nicotine, which is addictive and toxic to developing fetuses. Nicotine exposure can also harm adolescent and young adult brain development, which continues into the early to mid-20s. E-cigarette aerosol can contain chemicals that are harmful to the lungs. Youth e-cigarette use is associated with the use of other tobacco products, including cigarettes.

ARE E-CIGARETTES LESS HARMFUL THAN REGULAR CIGARETTES?

Yes, but that does not mean e-cigarettes are safe. E-cigarette aerosol generally contains fewer toxic chemicals than the deadly mix of 7,000 chemicals in smoke from regular cigarettes. However, e-cigarette aerosol is not harmless. It can contain harmful and potentially harmful substances, including nicotine, heavy metals such as lead, volatile organic compounds, and cancer-causing agents.

CAN E-CIGARETTES HELP ADULTS QUIT SMOKING CIGARETTES?

The FDA does not currently approve e-cigarettes as a quit-smoking aid. The U.S. Preventive Services Task Force (USPSTF), a group of health experts that makes recommendations about preventive health care, has concluded that evidence is insufficient to recommend e-cigarettes for smoking cessation in adults, including pregnant adults.

However, e-cigarettes may help nonpregnant adults who smoke if used as a complete substitute for all cigarettes and other smoked tobacco products.

To date, the few studies on the issue are mixed. A Cochrane Review found evidence from two randomized controlled trials that e-cigarettes with nicotine can help adults who smoke stop smoking in the long term compared with placebo (nonnicotine) e-cigarettes. However, there are some limitations to the existing research, including the small number of trials, small sample sizes, and wide margins of error around the estimates. A recent Centers for Disease Control and Prevention (CDC) study found that many adults are using e-cigarettes in an attempt to quit smoking. However, most adult e-cigarette users do not stop smoking cigarettes and instead continue to use both products (known as "dual use"). Dual use is not an effective way to safeguard your health, whether you are using e-cigarettes, smokeless tobacco, or other tobacco products in addition to regular cigarettes. Because smoking even a few cigarettes a day can be dangerous, quitting smoking completely is very important to protect your health.

WHO IS USING E-CIGARETTES?

E-cigarettes are the most commonly used tobacco product among youth.

- In 2023, 2.13 million U.S. middle and high school students used e-cigarettes in the past 30 days, including 4.6 percent of middle school students and 10.0 percent of high school students.

- In 2022, 2.55 million U.S. middle and high school students used e-cigarettes in the past 30 days, including 3.3 percent of middle school students and 14.1 percent of high school students.
- In 2021, 4.5 percent of U.S. adults currently used e-cigarettes.
- In 2019, among adults who currently used e-cigarettes overall, 36.9 percent also currently smoked cigarettes, 39.5 percent formerly smoked cigarettes, and 23.6 percent had never smoked cigarettes.
- Among adults who currently used e-cigarettes, the percentage who have never smoked cigarettes is highest among those aged 18–24 years (56.0%), and is lower in older age groups.[1]

Some people try to cut back on smoking cigarettes or work toward quitting smoking completely by using e-cigarettes, smokeless tobacco, or other tobacco products in addition to regular cigarettes. This is called "dual use." Dual use is not an effective way to safeguard health.

Because smoking even a few cigarettes a day can be dangerous, quitting smoking completely is very important to protect your health. If you have never smoked or used other tobacco products, including e-cigarettes, do not start.

HEALTH RISKS OF SMOKING

Smoking even a few cigarettes a day can be dangerous and can lead to serious health problems.

- People who smoke fewer than five cigarettes a day can have early signs of cardiovascular disease (CVD).
- Just cutting back on cigarettes may not protect someone from early death. People who smoke heavily and reduce their cigarette use by half still have a very

[1] "About E-cigarettes (Vapes)," Centers for Disease Control and Prevention (CDC), May 15, 2024. Available online. URL: www.cdc.gov/tobacco/e-cigarettes/about.html. Accessed July 22, 2024.

high risk of early death. On average, people who smoke die 10 years earlier than people who do not smoke.
- People who reported smoking in social situations rather than on a daily basis—a behavior referred to as "social smoking"—have similar blood pressure and cholesterol levels as people who smoke regularly.

QUITTING CAN IMPROVE YOUR HEALTH

Quitting smoking completely improves both your health and quality of life (QOL). This is true regardless of your age or how long you have been smoking.

When you quit smoking completely:

- After 1–2 years, your risk of heart attack drops sharply and continues to drop over time.
- After 5–10 years, your risk of stroke decreases.
- After 5 years, your risk for cancers of the mouth, throat, and voice box drops by half.
- After 10–15 years, your risk of lung cancer drops by half.

People who quit smoking completely live longer than those who keep smoking. The earlier you quit, the lower your risk for early death. Even quitting at age 50 cuts your risk in half for early death from a smoking-related disease.[2]

[2] "Dual Use of Tobacco Products," Centers for Disease Control and Prevention (CDC), October 13, 2023. Available online. URL: www.cdc.gov/tobacco/campaign/tips/diseases/dual-tobacco-use.html. Accessed April 9, 2024.

Chapter 5 | **Heated Tobacco Products**

Heated tobacco products heat processed tobacco leaf, allowing users to inhale nicotine into their lungs. Some brands of heated tobacco products permitted for sale in the United States include IQOS and Eclipse. More research is needed to understand the short- and long-term health effects of heated tobacco products.

The use of any type of tobacco product—including heated tobacco products—is harmful. They are especially harmful for youth, young adults, and pregnant women, as well as adults who do not currently use tobacco products. Heated tobacco products have not been scientifically shown to help smokers quit. If you have never used tobacco products, including heated tobacco products, do not start.

WHAT ARE HEATED TOBACCO PRODUCTS?

Sometimes marketed as "heat-not-burn" products, heated tobacco products come in many forms:

- Some use electronic heating elements.
- Some heat specially designed sticks, plugs, or capsules containing tobacco. This is how the electronically heated tobacco product authorized for sale in the United States works.
- Some work by heating liquids, creating an emission that passes through a tobacco plug to absorb flavor and nicotine from the tobacco.
- Some have a sealed part of the device that heats loose tobacco, either alone or together with flowers from the marijuana (cannabis) plant.

- Some are used with flavorings.
- Some allow users to control factors such as temperature.

Some heated tobacco products have a similar size and shape to regular cigarettes and have a carbon tip wrapped in glass fibers that the user heats with a lighter or match. Federal law allows this product to be sold in the United States.

ARE HEATED TOBACCO PRODUCTS THE SAME AS ELECTRONIC CIGARETTES?

No. Heated tobacco products heat actual tobacco leaves. In contrast, electronic cigarettes (e-cigarettes) heat liquids that typically contain nicotine derived from tobacco, as well as flavorings and other ingredients.

WHAT ARE THE HEALTH EFFECTS OF USING HEATED TOBACCO PRODUCTS?

Heated tobacco products are still new in the United States. Scientists are still learning about their short- and long-term health effects. The use of any tobacco product—including heated tobacco products—is harmful, especially for youth, young adults, and pregnant women. They are also harmful to adults who do not currently use tobacco products.

Regardless of whether they are heated by flame or electronically, heated tobacco products contain nicotine. Nicotine is highly addictive and can also harm the developing adolescent brain, which continues to develop until about age 25. Using nicotine in adolescence can harm the parts of the brain that control attention, learning, mood, and impulse control. It may also increase the risk of future addiction to other drugs. Nicotine is toxic to developing fetuses.

IS IT HARMFUL TO BREATHE THE SECONDHAND EMISSIONS FROM HEATED TOBACCO PRODUCTS?

Heated tobacco products produce emissions that are not as safe as clean air. Studies of secondhand emissions from heated tobacco products suggest that the products expose both users and bystanders to some of the same chemicals found in cigarette smoke, although at lower levels than cigarette smoke. Additional research is needed to understand the health effects of heated tobacco products and their emissions.

ARE HEATED TOBACCO PRODUCTS LESS HARMFUL THAN REGULAR CIGARETTES?

The emissions created from heated tobacco products generally contain lower levels of harmful ingredients than the smoke from regular cigarettes. However, this does not mean heated tobacco products are safe. Research suggests that heated tobacco products and their emissions contain many of the same harmful ingredients as regular cigarettes, as well as other harmful ingredients not present in regular cigarettes.

Additional research is needed to determine whether adult cigarette smokers who completely switch to heated tobacco products might reduce their risks of tobacco-related disease. Studies from other countries suggest that most adults who use heated tobacco products have not quit using cigarettes. Surveys of young adults in the United States suggest that young adults also use heated tobacco products in combination with other tobacco products. The use of multiple tobacco products is associated with an increased risk of nicotine dependence and adverse health effects.

As of February 2022, the U.S. Food and Drug Administration (FDA) has authorized only one heated tobacco product system (IQOS and three of its tobacco-containing Heatstick products) to be marketed as modified-risk tobacco products. These were the first tobacco products to receive "exposure modification" orders. These specific products may be marketed with claims that a person who uses regular cigarettes and fully switches to IQOS can reduce their exposure to harmful chemicals.

Similar claims may not be made about other heated tobacco products or about secondhand exposure to emissions from these products. In addition, the manufacturer of IQOS may not claim that using IQOS reduces the risk of disease, that the products are endorsed or approved by the FDA, or that the FDA deems the products to be safe for use by consumers.

WHO IS USING HEATED TOBACCO PRODUCTS?

These products are new in the United States. As of February 2022, the FDA has authorized only IQOS and Eclipse heated tobacco products for sale in this country. Sales of other heated tobacco products are growing worldwide.

The CDC began tracking the use of heated tobacco products among U.S. adults in 2017. At that time, 0.7 percent of adults, including 2.7 percent of people who currently smoked regular cigarettes, reported they had ever used a heated tobacco product. Reported use of heated tobacco products increased in 2018, when 2.4 percent of adults, including 6.7 percent of people who currently smoked regular cigarettes, reported to the CDC that they had ever used a heated tobacco product.

A different survey from 2019 found that the proportion of adults who use e-cigarettes and reported having ever used a heated tobacco product was higher than the proportion of adults who smoke cigarettes and reported having ever used a heated tobacco product. In 2023, 1.0 percent of U.S. middle and high school students combined reported having used heated tobacco products in the past 30 days.

WHAT CAN PEOPLE DO TO ADDRESS THE USE OF HEATED TOBACCO PRODUCTS?

- States, communities, tribes, and territories can implement evidence-based, population-level strategies that address the use of all forms of tobacco products, including heated tobacco products, such as:
  - incorporating all tobacco products, including heated tobacco products, into smoke-free and tobacco-free policies
  - licensing retailers who sell tobacco products, restricting young people's access to tobacco products in retail settings, and enforcing laws that penalize retailers who sell tobacco products to underage people
  - implementing policies to raise the price of tobacco products

    - reducing access to flavored tobacco products
    - curbing advertising and marketing for tobacco products that is appealing to young people
    - developing educational initiatives that warn about the risks of tobacco product use, especially among young people
- Parents and teachers can:
    - learn about the different types of tobacco products and the risks of using tobacco products, including heated tobacco products
    - set a good example by being tobacco-free and maintaining a tobacco-free home
    - talk to children, teens, and young adults about why all forms of tobacco products are harmful to them
    - develop, implement, and enforce tobacco-free school policies and prevention programs that are free from tobacco industry influence and that address all types of tobacco products, including heated tobacco products
- Health professionals can:
    - learn about the different types of tobacco products and the risks of using tobacco products
    - ask about the use of all forms of tobacco products, including heated tobacco products, when screening patients for the use of tobacco products
    - talk to children, teens, and young adults about why all forms of tobacco products are harmful to them
    - encourage patients to quit using tobacco products[1]

[1] "Heated Tobacco Products," Centers for Disease Control and Prevention (CDC), May 15, 2024. Available online. URL: www.cdc.gov/tobacco/other-tobacco-products/heated-tobacco-products.html. Accessed July 22, 2024.

Chapter 6 | **Smokeless Tobacco Products**

Chapter Contents

Section 6.1 | Chewing Tobacco, Snuff, and Snus

Smokeless tobacco is tobacco that is not burned or inhaled by the user. It is also known as "chewing tobacco," "chew," "dipping tobacco," "dip," "oral tobacco," "spit," "spitting tobacco," and "snuff." Most people chew or suck (dip) the tobacco in their mouth and spit out the tobacco juices that build up. There is also spitless smokeless tobacco.

TYPES OF SMOKELESS TOBACCO PRODUCTS

There are two main types of smokeless tobacco products:

- **Chewing tobacco.** Available as loose leaves, plugs (bricks), or twists of rope. A piece of tobacco is placed between the cheek and lower lip, typically near the back of the mouth. It is either chewed or held in place. Saliva is spit out or swallowed.
- **Snuff tobacco.** Finely cut or powdered tobacco. It is packaged moist or dry, with most American snuff being moist. Snuff may be sold in different scents and flavors. Dip or dipping tobacco and snus are common forms of moist snuff in the United States. It is available loose or in small pouches similar to tea bags. People take a pinch or pouch of moist snuff and put it between the cheek and gums—or behind the lips.

ARE CHEW AND DIP ADDICTIVE?

Yes. Both dip and chewing tobacco contain nicotine, which is addictive. People who use smokeless tobacco and people who smoke have similar levels of nicotine in their blood. With smokeless tobacco, nicotine is absorbed through the mouth and gets into the blood, then it goes to the brain. Even after people take tobacco out of their mouths, nicotine is still being absorbed into their blood. Research shows that nicotine stays in the blood longer for people who use smokeless tobacco than for people who smoke.

ARE CHEW AND DIP HARMFUL?

Yes—there are many harmful health effects of chewing tobacco and dip, including:

- **Cancer**. Smokeless tobacco has high levels of chemicals and other substances that can cause cancer, especially mouth and throat cancer. It can also cause leathery white patches in the mouth that can turn into cancer.
- **Tooth decay and mouth sores**. The sugar in smokeless tobacco can cause tooth decay and painful mouth sores.
- **Poor gum health**. Dip and chew can cause people's gums to pull away from their teeth, which can lead to loose teeth.[1]

Section 6.2 | Dissolvable Tobacco Products

Dissolvables are finely ground tobacco pressed into shapes such as tablets, sticks, or strips. These products slowly dissolve in the mouth and may appeal to youth because they come in attractive packaging, look like candy or small mints, and can be easily hidden from view.

TYPES OF DISSOLVABLE TOBACCO PRODUCTS

- **Lozenges**. Resemble pellets or tablets.
- **Orbs**. Resemble small mints.
- **Sticks**. Have a toothpick-like appearance.
- **Strips**. Thin sheets that work like dissolvable breath strips or medication strips.

MARKETING INFORMATION

Some cigarette companies make and sell smokeless tobacco products. In 2019, $576.1 million was spent on advertising and

[1] Smokefree Veterans, "Facts about Dipping and Chewing Tobacco," U.S. Department of Health and Human Services (HHS), January 22, 2024. Available online. URL: https://veterans.smokefree.gov/quit-dip-vapes/smokeless-tobacco/get-the-facts. Accessed April 9, 2024.

promotion of smokeless tobacco products, a decrease from 2018. Price discounts comprised nearly 65.3 percent of all advertising and promotion expenditures in 2019. Smokeless tobacco products include dry snuff, moist snuff, plug/twist, loose-leaf chewing tobacco, snus, and dissolvable products. Some cigarette companies advertise that smokeless tobacco can be used in places where tobacco smoking is not allowed. Additional research is needed to examine the long-term effects of newer smokeless tobacco products, such as dissolvables and U.S. snus.[1]

REPORTING A TOBACCO PRODUCT PROBLEM OR VIOLATION

If you have experienced undesired health or quality problems with any tobacco product, including dissolvable tobacco, you can report it to the U.S. Food and Drug Administration (FDA). Knowing more about adverse experiences can help the FDA identify concerning trends and causes or contributors for particular incidents or health or quality problems beyond those normally associated with tobacco product use. You can read some tobacco-related adverse experience reports on the Tobacco Product Problem Reports page (www.fda.gov/tobacco-products/tobacco-science-research/tobacco-product-problem-reports).

If you believe these products are being sold to minors, or you see another potential violation of the U.S. Federal Food, Drug, and Cosmetic Act (FD&C Act) or the FDA's tobacco regulations, report the potential violation.

FDA REGULATIONS FOR DISSOLVABLE TOBACCO PRODUCTS

The FDA regulates dissolvable tobacco products to ensure their safety and proper labeling. These regulations cover various aspects, including manufacturing, import, packaging, labeling, advertising, promotion, sale, and distribution.

[1] "Smokeless Tobacco: Products and Marketing," Centers for Disease Control and Prevention (CDC), May 14, 2021. Available online. URL: www.cdc.gov/tobacco/data_statistics/fact_sheets/smokeless/products_marketing/index.htm#not-burned. Accessed April 9, 2024.

Key Points to Know

- **Regulated by the FDA**. The FDA regulates dissolvable tobacco products under the FD&C Act. This regulation includes everything from how these products are made to how they are advertised and sold.
- **Therapeutic products**. If dissolvable tobacco products are marketed as a way to help people quit smoking, they are regulated by the FDA as drugs through the Center for Drug Evaluation and Research (CDER).
- **Manufacturing and importing**. If you are involved in making, modifying, mixing, assembling, processing, labeling, repacking, or importing tobacco products, you are considered a tobacco product manufacturer. This includes anyone who imports finished tobacco products.
- **Compliance information**. Manufacturers must follow specific FDA regulations. The FDA's Center for Tobacco Products (CTP) website provides more information on how to comply with these regulations.
- **Small business assistance**. The CTP's Office of Small Business Assistance can help answer questions about regulations and compliance for small businesses and provide educational resources to help them understand FDA regulations and policies.

For more detailed information and resources, visit the FDA's Center for Tobacco Products web page (www.fda.gov/tobacco-products/compliance-enforcement-training/manufacturing).[2]

[2] "Dissolvable Tobacco Products," U.S. Food and Drug Administration (FDA), August 22, 2023. Available online. URL: www.fda.gov/tobacco-products/products-ingredients-components/dissolvable-tobacco-products. Accessed April 9, 2024.

Chapter 7 | **Nontobacco Nicotine**

Nontobacco nicotine (NTN) refers to nicotine that does not come from a tobacco plant. NTN includes synthetic nicotine, made in a lab and has a similar molecular makeup as naturally occurring nicotine.

NICOTINE SOURCES

Nicotine is naturally present in tobacco plants. Most tobacco products, including cigarettes, cigars, and smokeless tobacco, contain nicotine derived from these plants. The e-liquid in electronic cigarettes (e-cigarettes) usually contains nicotine from tobacco. Recently, many companies, including manufacturers of popular youth e-cigarette brands, have started using NTN in their products.

IS NONTOBACCO NICOTINE ADDICTIVE?

Yes. Nicotine is addictive regardless of its source, including NTN. Tobacco products are addictive because they contain nicotine, which keeps people using these products even when they want to stop. No tobacco product is safe. Young people are at a higher risk of becoming addicted to nicotine in tobacco products than adults because their brains are still developing. Nicotine exposure during adolescence can disrupt normal brain development. If you are an adult who does not use tobacco products, you should stay tobacco-free. If you use tobacco products, resources are available to help you quit.

DOES THE FDA REGULATE NONTOBACCO NICOTINE PRODUCTS?

Yes, the U.S. Food and Drug Administration (FDA) regulates NTN products. Since the passage of the Family Smoking Prevention and

Tobacco Control Act (commonly called the "Tobacco Control Act") in 2009, the FDA has regulated the manufacturing, distribution, and marketing of tobacco products. In 2016, the Deeming Rule extended the FDA's authority to include more tobacco products, including e-cigarettes.

In response to the increase in NTN in popular tobacco products, Congress passed a federal law that went into effect on April 14, 2022, clarifying the FDA's authority to regulate tobacco products containing nicotine from any source, including synthetic nicotine. This law imposes requirements under the U.S. Federal Food, Drug, and Cosmetic Act (FD&C Act) for manufacturers, importers, retailers, and distributors of NTN products. Manufacturers of NTN products who wish to market their products must submit a premarket application and obtain FDA authorization, or they will be subject to FDA enforcement.

IS IT LEGAL TO SELL NONTOBACCO NICOTINE PRODUCTS?

Nontobacco nicotine products can only be legally marketed in the United States if they receive premarket authorization from the FDA. Without FDA marketing authorization, a product violates the FD&C Act and is subject to FDA enforcement. Manufacturers of NTN products are held to the same public health standards as other tobacco products. This includes requirements to prevent youth access to these products and the submission of a premarket application for FDA authorization to sell their products.

FDA REVIEW OF NONTOBACCO NICOTINE APPLICATIONS

A substantial number of applications were submitted by May 14, 2022—nearly 1 million from more than 200 separate companies. The FDA has been actively preparing for, processing, and reviewing these applications since the new law was passed. The FDA has completed an acceptance review of 100 percent of the NTN applications submitted by May 14, 2022, accepting over 9,500 applications, with the majority for e-cigarette or e-liquid products. Acceptance is not a determination of the product's authorization status; these applications will proceed to more substantial review. The FDA issued refuse-to-accept (RTA) letters for over 926,000 products in applications that do not meet the criteria for acceptance. As of October 2023, the FDA had made determinations on over 98 percent of the applications received. Currently, no NTN products have received marketing authorizations.

FDA ENFORCEMENT AGAINST ILLEGAL NONTOBACCO NICOTINE PRODUCTS

The FDA continues to pursue enforcement actions as swiftly as possible. Since Congress clarified the FDA's authority to regulate NTN products, the FDA has issued:

- warning letters to manufacturers, such as Puff Bar, a brand popular among youth
- warning letters to retailers for the sale of NTN products to underage purchasers
- civil money penalties for sales of NTN products to underage purchasers

Failure to promptly correct warning letter violations can result in further actions such as civil money penalties, seizure, and/or injunction.[1]

REQUIREMENTS FOR PRODUCTS MADE WITH NONTOBACCO NICOTINE

New legislation enacted on March 15, 2022, clarifies that the FDA can regulate tobacco products containing nicotine from any source. This law took effect on April 14, 2022. As of this date, manufacturers, distributors, importers, and retailers of tobacco products containing NTN—nicotine not made or derived from tobacco, such as synthetic nicotine—must ensure compliance with applicable requirements under the FD&C Act, such as:

- not selling these products to persons under 21 years of age (both in-person and online)

[1] "Requirements for Products Made with Nontobacco Nicotine Take Effect April 14," U.S. Food and Drug Administration (FDA), April 13, 2022. Available online. URL: www.fda.gov/tobacco-products/ctp-newsroom/requirements-products-made-non-tobacco-nicotine-take-effect-april-14. Accessed April 10, 2024.

- not marketing these products as modified-risk tobacco products without FDA authorization
- not distributing free samples of these products

Additionally, owners and operators of establishments engaged in the manufacture, preparation, compounding, or processing of NTN products must register with the FDA and list all tobacco products they manufacture, prepare, compound, or process for commercial distribution. Manufacturers of NTN products who wish to market their products must submit a premarket application and obtain FDA authorization, or they will be subject to FDA enforcement.

For more information on these regulations and how to comply, visit the FDA's Center for Tobacco Products (CTP) web page (www.fda.gov/tobacco-products/about-center-tobacco-products-ctp/contact-ctp).

FDA leaders have also authored an opinion piece on the legislation, describing how this new law closes a loophole and allows the FDA to use its authorities to protect public health from the harms of tobacco products, regardless of the source of nicotine.[2]

[2] "Regulation and Enforcement of Nontobacco Nicotine (NTN) Products," U.S. Food and Drug Administration (FDA), November 6, 2023. Available online. URL: www.fda.gov/tobacco-products/products-ingredients-components/regulation-and-enforcement-non-tobacco-nicotine-ntn-products. Accessed April 10, 2024.

Chapter 8 | **Understanding Nicotine Addiction**

Chapter Contents

WHAT IS NICOTINE?

Nicotine is the chemical found in tobacco products that is responsible for addiction. When you use tobacco, nicotine is quickly absorbed into your body and goes directly to your brain. Nicotine activates areas of the brain that make you feel satisfied and happy. Whether you smoke, vape, or dip, the nicotine you are putting in your body is dangerously addictive and can be harmful to your developing brain.[1]

HOW DOES NICOTINE WORK?

Nicotine is absorbed into your bloodstream and goes to your adrenal glands just above your kidneys. The glands release adrenaline, which increases your blood pressure, breathing, and heart rate. Adrenaline also gives you a lot of good feelings all at once.[2]

WHY IS NICOTINE DANGEROUS?

Nicotine can lead to addiction, which puts you at risk of becoming a lifelong smoker and exposing you to the many harmful chemicals in tobacco. These chemicals cause cancer and harm almost every organ in your body. Teens are especially sensitive to nicotine's addictive effects because their brains are still developing, which makes it easier to get hooked. Using nicotine at a young age can also rewire your brain to become more easily addicted to other drugs.

Nicotine can have other long-lasting effects on brain development, making it harder to concentrate, learn, and control impulses.[3]

---

[1] Smokefree Teen, "Nicotine and Addiction," U.S. Department of Health and Human Services (HHS), September 15, 2017. Available online. URL: https://teen.smokefree.gov/the-risks-of-tobacco/nicotine-addiction. Accessed April 9, 2024.

[2] "Mind Matters: The Body's Response to Nicotine, Tobacco and Vaping," National Institute on Drug Abuse (NIDA), November 1, 2019. Available online. URL: https://nida.nih.gov/research-topics/parents-educators/lesson-plans/mind-matters/nicotine-tobacco-vaping. Accessed April 9, 2024.

[3] See footnote [1].

HOW DO YOU BECOME ADDICTED TO NICOTINE?

Over time, the nicotine in tobacco can change the way your brain works. If you stop using it, your body can get confused, and you can start to feel really sick. This makes it hard to stop using these products even when you know they are bad for you.[4]

Addiction is characterized by compulsive drug-seeking and use, even in the face of negative health consequences. The majority of smokers would like to stop smoking, and each year about half try to quit permanently. Yet, only about 6 percent of smokers are able to quit in a given year. Most smokers will need to make multiple attempts before they are able to quit permanently. Medications, including varenicline, some antidepressants (e.g., bupropion), and nicotine-replacement therapy (NRT), can help in many cases.

The Effect of Nicotine on the Brain

A transient surge of endorphins in the reward circuits of the brain causes a slight, brief euphoria when nicotine is administered. This surge is much briefer than the high associated with other drugs. However, like other drugs of abuse, nicotine increases levels of the neurotransmitter dopamine in these reward circuits, which reinforces the behavior of taking the drug. Repeated exposure alters these circuits' sensitivity to dopamine and leads to changes in other brain circuits involved in learning, stress, and self-control. For many tobacco users, the long-term brain changes induced by continued nicotine exposure result in addiction, which involves withdrawal symptoms when not smoking and difficulty adhering to the resolution to quit.

Nicotine's Addictive Properties

The pharmacokinetic properties of nicotine, or the way it is processed by the body, contribute to its addictiveness. When cigarette smoke enters the lungs, nicotine is absorbed rapidly in the blood and delivered quickly to the brain, so that nicotine levels peak within 10 seconds of inhalation. But the acute effects of nicotine also dissipate quickly, along with the associated feelings of reward;

---

[4] See footnote [2].

this rapid cycle causes the smoker to continue dosing to maintain the drug's pleasurable effects and prevent withdrawal symptoms.

Withdrawal and Its Effects

Withdrawal occurs as a result of dependence, when the body becomes used to having the drug in the system. Being without nicotine for too long can cause a regular user to experience irritability, craving, depression, anxiety, cognitive and attention deficits, sleep disturbances, and increased appetite. These withdrawal symptoms may begin within a few hours after the last cigarette, quickly driving people back to tobacco use.

When a person quits smoking, withdrawal symptoms peak within the first few days of the last cigarette smoked and usually subside within a few weeks. For some people, however, symptoms may persist for months, and the severity of withdrawal symptoms appears to be influenced by a person's genes.

Cognitive and Behavioral Effects of Nicotine

In addition to its pleasurable effects, nicotine also temporarily boosts aspects of cognition, such as the ability to sustain attention and hold information in memory. However, long-term smoking is associated with cognitive decline and the risk of Alzheimer disease (AD), suggesting that short-term nicotine-related enhancement does not outweigh long-term consequences for cognitive functioning. In addition, people in withdrawal from nicotine experience neurocognitive deficits such as problems with attention or memory. These neurocognitive withdrawal symptoms are increasingly recognized as a contributor to continued smoking. A small research study also suggested that withdrawal may impair sleep for severely dependent smokers, which may additionally contribute to relapse.

Environmental and Behavioral Triggers

In addition to the drug's effect on multiple neurotransmitters and their receptors, many behavioral factors can affect the severity of withdrawal symptoms. For many people who smoke, the feel, smell, and sight of a cigarette and the ritual of obtaining, handling, lighting, and smoking the cigarette are all associated with the pleasurable effects of smoking and can make withdrawal or craving worse. Learning processes in the brain associate these cues with nicotine-induced dopamine surges in the reward system, similar to what occurs with other drug addictions.

COPING WITH NICOTINE ADDICTION

Nicotine replacement therapies such as gum, patches, and inhalers, and other medications approved for the treatment of nicotine addiction may help alleviate the physiological aspects of withdrawal; however, cravings often persist because of the power of these cues. Behavioral therapies can help smokers identify environmental triggers of cravings, so they can use strategies to avoid these triggers and manage the feelings that arise when triggers cannot be avoided.[5]

Section 8.2 | **Genetics of Nicotine Dependence**

New scientific developments can improve our understanding of nicotine addiction and spur the development of better prevention and treatment strategies.

GENETICS AND EPIGENETICS

An estimated 50–75 percent of the risk for nicotine addiction is attributable to genetic factors. A cluster of genes (*CHRNA5-CHRNA3-CHRNB4*) on chromosome 15, which encode the $\alpha 5$, $\alpha 3$, and $\beta 4$ protein subunits that make up the brain receptor for nicotine, are particularly implicated in nicotine dependence and smoking among people of European descent. Variation in the *CHRNA5* gene influences the effectiveness of combination

[5] "Is Nicotine Addictive?" National Institute on Drug Abuse (NIDA), May 1, 2022. Available online. URL: https://nida.nih.gov/publications/research-reports/tobacco-nicotine-e-cigarettes/nicotine-addictive. Accessed April 9, 2024.

nicotine replacement therapy (NRT), but not varenicline. Other research has identified genes that influence nicotine metabolism and, therefore, the number of cigarettes smoked, responsiveness to medication, and chances of successfully quitting. For example, the therapeutic response to varenicline is associated with variants in the *CHRNB2*, *CHRNA5*, and *CHRNA4* genes, while bupropion-related cessation is linked with variation in genes that affect nicotine metabolism.

Smoking can also lead to persistent changes in gene expression (epigenetic changes), which may contribute to associated medical consequences over the long term, even following cessation. Epigenetic changes may serve as a potential biomarker for prenatal tobacco smoke exposure. Researchers found tobacco-specific changes at 26 sites on the epigenome, and this pattern predicted prenatal exposure with 81 percent accuracy. A large-scale meta-analysis of data on epigenetic changes associated with prenatal exposure to cigarette smoke also identified many epigenetic changes that persisted into later childhood. More research is needed to understand the long-term health effects of these changes.

NEUROIMAGING

Cutting-edge neuroimaging technologies have identified brain changes associated with nicotine dependence and smoking. Using functional magnetic resonance imaging (fMRI), scientists can visualize smokers' brains as they respond to cigarette-associated cues that can trigger craving and relapse. Such research may lead to a biomarker for relapse risk and for monitoring treatment progress, as well as point to regions of the brain involved in the development of nicotine addiction.

A neuroimaging technology called "default-mode" or "resting-state fMRI" (rs-fMRI) reveals intrinsic brain activity when people are alert but not performing a particular task. Using this technique, researchers are examining the neurobiological profile associated with withdrawal and how nicotine affects cognition. Comparisons between smokers and nonsmokers suggest that chronic nicotine may weaken connectivity within brain circuits involved in planning, paying attention, and behavioral control—possibly contributing to difficulty with quitting. fMRI studies also reveal the effect of smoking cessation medications on the brain—particularly how they modulate the activity of different brain regions to alleviate withdrawal symptoms and reduce smoking. A review of these studies suggested that NRT enhances cognition during withdrawal by modulating activity in default-network regions, but may not affect neural circuits associated with nicotine addiction.

Some imaging techniques allow researchers to visualize neurotransmitters and their receptors, further informing our understanding of nicotine addiction and its treatment. Using these techniques, researchers have established that smoking increases the number of brain receptors for nicotine. Individuals who show greater receptor upregulation are less likely to stop smoking. Combining neuroimaging and genetics may yield useful information for improving and tailoring treatment. For example, nonsmoking adolescents with a particular variant in the *CHRNA5-CHRNA3-CHRNB4* gene cluster (which is associated with nicotine dependence and smoking) showed reduced brain activity in response to reward in the striatum as well as the orbitofrontal and anterior cingulate cortex. This finding suggests that genetics can influence how the brain processes rewards, which may influence vulnerability to nicotine dependence. Neuroimaging genetics also shows that other genes, including ones that influence dopamine neurotransmission, influence reward sensitivity and risk for addiction to nicotine.[1]

RESEARCHERS FIND GENETIC VULNERABILITY TO MENTHOL CIGARETTE USE

A study funded by the U.S. Food and Drug Administration (FDA) and the National Institutes of Health (NIH) found an unexpected sensory variant exclusive to African Americans.

A genetic variant found only in people of African descent significantly increases a smoker's preference for cigarettes containing

[1] "What Research Is Being Done on Tobacco Use?" National Institute on Drug Abuse (NIDA), May 1, 2022. Available online. URL: https://nida.nih.gov/publications/research-reports/tobacco-nicotine-e-cigarettes/what-research-being-done-tobacco-use. Accessed April 10, 2024.

menthol, a flavor additive. The variant of the *MRGPRX4* gene is five to eight times more frequent among smokers who use menthol cigarettes than other smokers, according to an international group of researchers supported by the FDA and the NIH. The multiethnic study is the first to examine all genes to identify genetic vulnerability to menthol cigarettes. The paper was published online in the journal *Public Library of Science* (*PLOS*) *Genetics* on February 15.

Menthol provides a minty taste and a cooling or soothing sensation and plays a particularly troubling role in U.S. cigarette smoking patterns. According to the FDA, nearly 20 million people in the United States smoke menthol cigarettes, which are particularly popular among African-American smokers and teen smokers. In the United States, 86 percent of African-American smokers use menthol cigarettes, compared to less than 30 percent of smokers of European descent. In addition, menthol cigarettes may be harder to quit than other cigarettes.

Although not originally the focus of the study, researchers also uncovered clues as to how menthol may reduce the irritation and harshness of smoking cigarettes.

THE MOLECULAR MECHANISMS OF MENTHOL INTERACTION

"This study sheds light on the molecular mechanisms of how menthol interacts with the body," said Andrew Griffith, MD, PhD, scientific director and acting deputy director of NIH's National Institute on Deafness and Other Communications Disorders (NIDCD). "These results can help inform public health strategies to lower the rates of harmful cigarette smoking among groups particularly vulnerable to using menthol cigarettes."

The research team, led by Dennis Drayna, PhD, chief of the Section on Genetics of Communication Disorders at the NIDCD, conducted detailed genetic analyses on 1,300 adults. In the initial analyses, researchers at the University of Texas Southwestern Medical Center, Dallas (UT Southwestern), used data from a multiethnic, population-based group of smokers from the Dallas Heart Study and from an African-American group of smokers from the Dallas Biobank. In conjunction with researchers from the Schroeder Institute for Tobacco Research, Washington, DC, the scientists further confirmed their findings in a group of African-American smokers enrolled in the Washington, DC, Tobacco Quitline.

The researchers report that 5–8 percent of the African-American study participants had the gene variant. None of the participants of European, Asian, or Native American descent had the variant.

Identifying the genetic variant pointed the researchers in an unexpected direction, leading them to provide the first characterization of this naturally occurring *MRGPRX4* variant in humans. The gene codes for a sensor, or receptor, that is believed to be involved in detecting and responding to irritants from the environment in the lungs and airways.

"We expected to find genes that relate to taste receptors, since menthol is a flavor additive," said Drayna. "Instead, we discovered a different kind of signaling molecule that appears to be involved in menthol preference."

Collaborators at the University of North Carolina (UNC), Chapel Hill, then worked with the research team to look more closely at the effect of the African-specific variant on the function of the *MRGPRX4* receptor. They found that the variant alters a specific type of cell signaling, and menthol further alters this. Additional studies confirmed that this sensor is found in the airways, suggesting that menthol is likely to affect how we sense irritation in the airways.

"While this gene variant cannot explain all of the increased use of menthol cigarettes by African Americans, our findings indicate that this variant is a potentially important factor that underlies the preference for menthol cigarettes in this population. While things such as cultural factors or industry advertising practices have been a focus for understanding menthol use thus far, our findings indicate that African-specific genetic factors also need to be considered," said Drayna.

IMPLICATIONS FOR PUBLIC HEALTH AND MENTHOL REGULATION

The FDA has sought public commentary and scientific information on the use of menthol in tobacco products. The agency has announced plans to propose a ban on menthol-flavored cigarettes and cigars, in large part because of the high use of menthol cigarettes among youth and young adults. More than half of smokers aged 12–17 smoke menthol-flavored cigarettes. The prevalence rises to 7 out of 10 among African-American youth who smoke, according to the FDA.[2]

---

[2] "Researchers Find Genetic Vulnerability to Menthol Cigarette Use," National Institutes of Health (NIH), February 15, 2019. Available online. URL: www.nih.gov/news-events/news-releases/researchers-find-genetic-vulnerability-menthol-cigarette-use. Accessed April 10, 2024.

Chapter 9 | **Influence of Cigarette Marketing on Youth Smoking**

THE CHALLENGE OF ETHICAL RESEARCH

The most definitive evidence of the influence of cigarette marketing on youth smoking would involve experimental manipulation of adolescents' long-term exposure to cigarette marketing and assessment of its effect on adolescents' initiation of smoking. However, such a study would be either unethical or unfeasible. Nevertheless, a body of experimental evidence exists about the effect of brief exposure to cigarette marketing on images of smokers, perceptions about the prevalence of smoking among adolescents, and intentions to smoke. Further, an abundance of evidence from multiple lines of research using other study designs collectively establishes a causal link between tobacco marketing and smoking behavior.

ADOLESCENT PSYCHOLOGICAL NEEDS

One type of evidence involves adolescent psychological needs. Many adolescents are motivated to smoke by the perception that doing so will help fulfill important psychological needs. Adolescents perceive that smoking will contribute to popularity and that advertising conveys this message. Those who believe the message are more likely to smoke. In addition, tobacco company documents show that marketing for cigarette brands popular with youth associates smoking those brands with popularity.

Many adolescents perceive that smoking will confer attributes associated with success with the opposite sex—toughness in the case of boys and slenderness in the case of girls. Girls are more likely to smoke if they think it will help them be thin and attractive. Cigarette marketing conveys that young women who smoke are high in sex appeal. Tobacco company documents show that several of the most youth-popular brands have been consistently and effectively associated with an image of rugged masculinity and sex appeal.

Many adolescents have a need to be rebellious and see smokers as having this characteristic. As a result, rebelliousness is a predictor of smoking initiation.

Adolescents' needs for sensation, risk-taking, and fun are also associated with smoking. Adolescents high in sensation seeking are more likely to smoke. Cigarette marketing frequently associates smoking with themes of fun and excitement. Many adolescents feel that cigarette advertising conveys that smokers will derive pleasure from smoking.

Cigarette marketing also exploits adolescents' needs to cope with depression and anxiety. Many adolescents perceive that smoking can help reduce distress. Adolescents high in stress or depression appear more likely to smoke. Those who are depressed and receptive to cigarette advertising are particularly vulnerable to initiating smoking. Numerous tobacco company documents indicate that cigarette marketing often conveys that smoking youth-popular brands will help a person to relax or better cope with stress.

CIGARETTE MARKETING AND IMAGE ENHANCEMENT

Because of the importance of popularity and peer acceptance in adolescence, most teenagers have a strong need for a positive self-image. Many adolescents perceive smokers to have a number of desirable traits. The perception that smoking will reinforce a desired self-image motivates those adolescents to smoke.

Both correlational and experimental studies show that exposure to cigarette marketing influences adolescents to have a more favorable image of smokers, to perceive that smoking among adolescents is more prevalent, and to have more positive intentions to smoke. The experimental studies provide particularly strong evidence of the influence of marketing. They control for other possible influences on smoking and rule out the possibility that there is a relationship between smoking and exposure to advertising simply because both are due to some third variable, such as innate curiosity about smoking.

EXPOSURE TO CIGARETTE MARKETING AND SMOKING SUSCEPTIBILITY AND BEHAVIOR

The longitudinal studies provide strong evidence of such an effect since exposure to tobacco marketing occurs before changes in smoking behavior occur. The findings are robust and consistent. In the overwhelming majority of studies, exposure to cigarette marketing was associated with smoking behavior. This was true for diverse measures of exposure, including self-reported exposure to advertisements, derived estimates of adolescents' exposure, recall of specific advertisements, recognition of brands in advertisements in which brand information had been removed, a variety of attitudes toward the advertisements, beliefs about the effect of advertising, and multicomponent indices of adolescents' receptivity to cigarette advertising. Measures of exposure predicted both increases in adolescents' stated intentions to smoke and the actual initiation of smoking.

Tobacco companies have repeatedly asserted that peer and family influences—not their marketing practices—influence adolescents to smoke. However, many of these cross-sectional and longitudinal studies of the influence of marketing exposure measured and analyzed social influences along with tobacco marketing exposure. They generally found that marketing practices influence adolescent smoking even after controlling for peer and parental influences. Indeed, a number of studies that used advertising and influence of peers and parents to predict later smoking or intent to smoke found that advertising exposure is a stronger predictor than peer or parental smoking.

These studies likely underestimate the influence of marketing practices, since some marketing influence develops through peers and parents. For example, tobacco companies design marketing to influence the perception that popular people smoke specific brands. These practices influence not just one person, but entire peer groups. Because of exposure to these advertisements, some adolescent peer groups may view smoking as the "in" thing. These groups are then more likely to approve and admire someone who smokes a brand that marketing tells them "in" people smoke.

Thus, evidence that an adolescent is more likely to smoke if his or her friends smoke is, in part, due to the influence cigarette marketing has on the entire peer group. Advertising that associates a cigarette brand with popularity prepares an entire peer group to approve of those who smoke it.

EFFECTS OF TOBACCO ADVERTISING ON TOBACCO CONSUMPTION

The issues and studies relative to this line of evidence indicate, at a minimum, that empirical estimation of the effects of tobacco advertising on tobacco consumption is a complex challenge. The most potentially valid econometric strategies are either cross-sectional data with advertising measured by independent sources at a local level or international data on comprehensive advertising bans. Many econometric studies use small samples of highly aggregated national time-series data and find little or no effect of advertising. This is because the advertising data employed have little variance and are measured at a level of expenditure at which advertising has little or no marginal effect. However, a meta-analysis that pooled the results of 24 such studies did find a small, but statistically significant, positive effect of advertising on cigarette consumption. The evidence from cross-sectional studies using disaggregated local-level data does indicate an effect of advertising on consumption. These time series and cross-sectional studies support the theory that the industry response function slopes upward and is subject to diminishing marginal effects.

The studies of advertising bans suggest that bans can reduce consumption under certain circumstances. Banning advertising in a limited number of media has little or no effect. Limited advertising bans do not reduce the total level of advertising expenditure but simply result in substitution to the remaining nonbanned media or to other marketing activities. Banning advertising in most or all available media can reduce tobacco consumption, because, in these circumstances, the possibilities for substitution to other media are limited.

CONCLUSIONS

- Much tobacco advertising targets the psychological needs of adolescents, such as popularity, peer acceptance, and positive self-image. Advertising creates the perception that smoking will satisfy these needs.
- Adolescents who believe that smoking can satisfy their psychological needs or whose desired image of themselves is similar to their image of smokers are more likely to smoke cigarettes.
- Experimental studies show that even brief exposure to tobacco advertising influences adolescents' attitudes and perceptions about smoking and smokers, and adolescents' intentions to smoke.
- The vast majority of cross-sectional studies find an association between exposure to cigarette advertising, measured in numerous ways, and adolescent smoking behavior, measured in numerous ways, indicating a robust association.
- Strong and consistent evidence from longitudinal studies indicates that exposure to cigarette advertising influences nonsmoking adolescents to initiate smoking and to move toward regular smoking.
- Many econometric studies have used national time-series data to examine the association between tobacco advertising expenditures and tobacco consumption. Some of these studies found a small positive effect of advertising on consumption. Other studies failed to find a positive effect, probably because the data used had little variance and were measured at a high level of advertising expenditure at which changes in the volume of advertising have little or no marginal effect.
- The evidence from three cross-sectional econometric studies using disaggregated local-level data indicates a positive effect of advertising on tobacco consumption.
- Studies of tobacco advertising bans in various countries show that comprehensive bans reduce tobacco consumption. Noncomprehensive restrictions generally

induce an increase in expenditures for advertising in nonbanned media and for other marketing activities, which offsets the effect of the partial ban so that any net change in consumption is minimal or undetectable.
- The total weight of evidence from multiple types of studies, conducted by investigators from different disciplines, using data from many countries, demonstrates a causal relationship between tobacco advertising and promotion and increased tobacco use, as manifested by increased smoking initiation and increased per capita tobacco consumption in the population.[1]

[1] Division of Cancer Control and Population Sciences (DCCPS), "Influence of Tobacco Marketing on Smoking Behavior," National Cancer Institute (NCI), June 2008. Available online. URL: https://cancercontrol.cancer.gov/sites/default/files/2020-06/m19_7.pdf. Accessed April 10, 2024.

Chapter 10 | **Addressing Health Inequities in Tobacco Use**

HEALTH EQUITY AND TOBACCO USE

Health equity is the fair and just opportunity for all people to be as healthy as possible, including the opportunity to be free from commercial tobacco*. However, some people do not have this opportunity due to factors such as race or ethnicity, where they live, or the type of job they have.

* *"Commercial tobacco" refers to harmful products made and sold by tobacco companies. It does not include "traditional tobacco" used by Indigenous groups for religious or ceremonial purposes.*

TARGETED MARKETING AND ITS INFLUENCE

For decades, tobacco companies have used promotions, targeted marketing, and other tactics to unfairly increase the access to and appeal of tobacco products for certain population groups. Discrimination, poverty, and other social conditions are linked to tobacco use and make quitting more difficult. These factors contribute to high levels of disease, disability, and death from tobacco use in some populations, such as Hispanic and Latinx people and those with behavioral health conditions.

More protections are needed to prevent tobacco use and secondhand smoke exposure among different population groups and to help people quit for good. Everyone deserves to be as healthy as possible, which means living free from the harmful effects of commercial tobacco. By increasing efforts in these areas, we can advance health equity.

SOCIAL DETERMINANTS OF HEALTH AND THEIR RELATIONSHIP TO HEALTH BEHAVIORS

Social determinants of health are conditions where people live, learn, work, and play that affect health and quality of life (QOL). Examples related to tobacco include the number of stores that sell tobacco in a neighborhood and where in stores tobacco products are displayed and advertised.

- **Education, job opportunities, and income**. Lower-quality education can be associated with a less ability to understand and act on health information and less access to good jobs with health insurance. People with lower incomes can have less access to health care, including care needed for smoking-related health conditions.
- **Stress**. Some social determinants of health can lead to stress, which can also affect tobacco use. Stress from financial problems, discrimination, or unsafe neighborhoods can make it harder to quit smoking and can increase tobacco use. Prolonged stress can lead to health problems such as high blood pressure (HBP) and type 2 diabetes.

TARGETED MARKETING OF COMMERCIAL TOBACCO PRODUCTS

Tobacco companies spend billions of dollars each year marketing their products, targeting specific population groups, including youth and people who are African American, Hispanic, American Indian and Alaska Native, Asian, LGBTQ+, and those in low-income communities.

- **Marketing tactics**. Promotions, scholarships, giveaways, nightlife marketing, price promotions, product placement, and event sponsorships are common tactics for targeting these groups.
- **Influence**. Tobacco product marketing can make smoking seem more appealing and increase the likelihood that someone will try smoking for the first time or start using tobacco products regularly.

ACTIONS TO IMPROVE TOBACCO-RELATED HEALTH INEQUITIES

States and communities can take action to make tobacco products less appealing and less available. Examples include:

- increasing prices and prohibiting price discounts
- prohibiting the sale of flavored tobacco products
- allowing fewer stores in a neighborhood to sell commercial tobacco products
- creating stronger smoke-free air policies that protect all people from secondhand smoke
- educating people about the dangers of exposure to secondhand smoke
- encouraging smoke-free environments in homes and vehicles
- keeping tobacco prices high
- reducing or eliminating the sale of tobacco products

ACCESS TO QUIT-SMOKING TREATMENT

Proven treatments, such as U.S. Food and Drug Administration (FDA)-approved medicines and behavioral counseling, can help people successfully quit smoking. However, some people face barriers to these treatments due to their location, employment status, or health insurance coverage. Barriers can also be related to race or culture.

To improve access to treatments, states, communities, and health-care systems can:

- ensure barrier-free health insurance coverage for evidence-based quit-smoking treatments
- integrate clinical screening and treatment for commercial tobacco use in all health-care settings
- increase access to quit-smoking services that are culturally acceptable and communicated in different languages
- share health messages that reach specific groups experiencing health disparities

BETTER HEALTH FOR ALL

A commitment to health equity involves understanding the causes of tobacco-related health disparities. By addressing social determinants of health, targeted marketing, and barriers to health care, states and communities can move toward health equity and reduce health disparities.[1]

[1] "Improving Tobacco-Related Health Disparities," Centers for Disease Control and Prevention (CDC), August 31, 2022. Available online. URL: www.cdc.gov/tobacco/tobacco-features/health-equity.html. Accessed July 21, 2024.

Chapter 11 | **Gender Differences in Tobacco Smoking**

Generally, men tend to use all tobacco products at higher rates than women. In 2015, 16.7 percent of adult males and 13.6 percent of adult females smoked cigarettes. These differences may relate to a combination of physiological factors (particularly ovarian hormones), cultural factors, and behavioral factors.

NEUROIMAGING FINDINGS

Results from neuroimaging studies suggest that smoking activates men's reward pathways more than women's. This finding is consistent with the idea that men smoke for the reinforcing effects of nicotine, whereas women smoke to regulate mood or in response to cigarette-related cues. A study of stress responses and cravings among male and female smokers trying to quit found that during abstinence, lower levels of the stress hormone cortisol predicted relapse in men. However, high cortisol levels were predictive of relapse in women. Other research on abstinence found that smoking a cigarette with nicotine, as compared to a denicotinized cigarette, alleviated withdrawal symptoms and negative mood to a greater extent in men than women. Women obtained equal relief from cigarettes with and without nicotine, suggesting that they found the drug less rewarding than men.

CIGARETTE CRAVING AND STRESS

Cigarette craving is a major reason why smokers find it hard to quit, and this strong urge to smoke can be evoked by sensory cues and stress. Research suggests that women experience stronger cravings than men in response to stress, but men may be more responsive to environmental cues. Additionally, longitudinal data from international surveys conducted in four industrialized countries indicated that men and women did not differ in their desire to quit, plans to quit, or quit attempts. However, women were 31 percent less likely to quit successfully. One reason women may have difficulty quitting is post-cessation weight gain. This concern should be addressed in behavioral counseling and adjunct treatments for all smokers.

MEDICATION EFFICACY

The overall lower cessation rate for women may reflect sex differences in response to particular medications. For example, varenicline has greater short- and immediate-term efficacy (at three and six months) among women smokers. However, women and men show similar one-year quit rates when using varenicline. In contrast, a combination of varenicline plus bupropion was less effective for cessation among women compared with men.

SMOKING DURING PREGNANCY

Another particular concern related to tobacco use among women is smoking during pregnancy. This issue requires targeted interventions to protect both maternal and fetal health.

By addressing these gender differences, health-care providers can develop more effective strategies for helping both men and women quit smoking.[1]

[1] "Are There Gender Differences in Tobacco Smoking?" National Institute on Drug Abuse (NIDA), May 1, 2022. Available online. URL: https://nida.nih.gov/publications/research-reports/tobacco-nicotine-e-cigarettes/are-there-gender-differences-in-tobacco-smoking. Accessed April 10, 2024.

Chapter 12 | **Smoking and Tobacco Use Demographics**

Chapter Contents

Section 12.1 | Youth and Tobacco Use

Youth use of tobacco products in any form is unsafe. Preventing tobacco product use among youth is critical to reducing tobacco use among the nation's youth.

Tobacco product use is started and established primarily during adolescence. Nearly 9 out of 10 adults who smoke cigarettes daily first try smoking by age 18. Flavorings in tobacco products can make them more appealing to youth. In 2021, 80.2 percent of high school students and 74.6 percent of middle school students who used tobacco products in the past 30 days reported using a flavored tobacco product during that time. In 2023, 90.3 percent of high school students and 87.1 percent of middle school students who used e-cigarettes in the past 30 days reported using a flavored e-cigarette during that time.

ESTIMATES OF CURRENT TOBACCO USE AMONG YOUTH

Electronic Cigarettes (E-cigarettes)

- E-cigarettes have been the most commonly used tobacco product among youth since 2014.
- In 2023, about 1 out of every 22 middle school students (4.6 percent) reported that they had used e-cigarettes in the past 30 days.
- In 2023, 1 of every 10 high school students (10.0 percent) reported that they had used e-cigarettes in the past 30 days.

Cigarettes

- In 2023, about 1 of every 100 middle school students (1.1 percent) reported that they had smoked cigarettes in the past 30 days.
- In 2023, nearly 2 of every 100 high school students (1.9 percent) reported that they had smoked cigarettes in the past 30 days.

Cigars

- In 2023, nearly 1 of every 100 middle school students (1.1 percent) reported that they had smoked cigars in the past 30 days.
- In 2023, nearly 2 of every 100 high school students (1.8 percent) reported that they had smoked cigars in the past 30 days.

Smokeless Tobacco

- In 2023, nearly 1 of every 100 middle school students (0.7 percent) reported that they had used smokeless tobacco in the past 30 days.
- In 2023, nearly 2 of every 100 high school students (1.5 percent) reported that they had used smokeless tobacco in the past 30 days.

Hookah

- In 2023, less than 1 of every 100 middle school students (1.0 percent) reported that they had smoked hookah in the past 30 days.
- In 2023, about 1 of every 100 high school students (1.1 percent) reported that they had smoked hookah in the past 30 days.

Heated Tobacco Products

- In 2023, less than 1 of every 100 middle school students (0.8 percent) and about 1 of every 100 high school students (1.0 percent) reported using heated tobacco products in the past 30 days.
- Heated tobacco products, also known as "heat-not-burn products," deliver nicotine to the user by heating tobacco leaves rather than a nicotine-containing liquid such as e-cigarettes.

Nicotine Pouches

- In 2023, about 1 of every 100 high school students (1.7 percent) reported using nicotine pouches in the past 30 days.

- Nicotine pouches are microfiber pouches with flavored nicotine powder that users dissolve in the mouth without spitting. Sales of nicotine pouches have increased rapidly in the United States.

All Tobacco Products Use

- In 2023, more than 6 of every 100 middle school students (6.6 percent) and about 1 of every 8 high school students (12.6 percent) reported current use of a tobacco product.
- In 2023, nearly 15 of every 100 middle school students (14.7 percent) and nearly 28 of every 100 high school students (27.9 percent) said they had ever tried a tobacco product.

Many Young People Use Multiple Tobacco Products

- In 2023, more than 2 of every 100 middle school students (2.5 percent) and about 1 of every 30 high school students (3.9 percent) reported current use of multiple tobacco products in the past 30 days.
- In 2023, about 6 of every 100 middle school students (6.1 percent) and more than 12 of every 100 high school students (12.7 percent) reported they had ever tried multiple tobacco products.

Youth who use multiple tobacco products are at higher risk for developing nicotine dependence and might be more likely to continue using tobacco into adulthood.

Table 12.1 explains the percentage of tobacco product use among high school students in 2023.

Table 12.1. Tobacco Product Use* among High School Students in 2023

Tobacco Product	Overall (%)	Girls (%)	Boys (%)
Any tobacco product†	12.60	14.10	11.20
Electronic cigarettes	10.00	12.20	8.00
Cigarettes	1.90	1.50	2.30

Table 12.1. Continued

Tobacco Product	Overall (%)	Girls (%)	Boys (%)
Cigars	1.80	1.40	2.30
Smokeless tobacco	1.50	–	2.10
Hookah	1.10	1.40	0.90
Nicotine pouches	1.70	–	2.60
Heated tobacco products	1.00	0.70	1.40
Pipe tobacco	0.60	0.50	0.70

** "Current use" is determined by respondents indicating that they have used a tobacco product on at least 1 day during the past 30 days.*
† In 2023, any tobacco product includes e-cigarettes, cigarettes, cigars, smokeless tobacco (composite), pipe tobacco, bidis (small brown cigarettes wrapped in a leaf), hookahs, heated tobacco products, nicotine pouches, and other oral nicotine products.

Table 12.2 explains the percentage of tobacco product use among middle school students in 2023.

Table 12.2. Tobacco Product Use* among Middle School Students in 2023

Tobacco Product	Overall (%)	Girls (%)	Boys (%)
Any tobacco product†	6.60	7.50	5.70
Electronic cigarettes	4.60	5.60	3.50
Cigarettes	1.10	1.10	–
Cigars	1.10	1.20	1.00
Smokeless tobacco	0.70	0.60	–
Hookah	1.00	–	0.80
Nicotine pouches	–	–	–
Heated tobacco products	0.80	0.80	–
Pipe tobacco	0.40	–	–

** "Current use" is determined by respondents indicating that they have used a tobacco product on at least 1 day during the past 30 days.*
† In 2023, any tobacco product includes e-cigarettes, cigarettes, cigars, smokeless tobacco (composite), pipe tobacco, bidis (small brown cigarettes wrapped in a leaf), hookahs, heated tobacco products, nicotine pouches, and other oral nicotine products.

FACTORS ASSOCIATED WITH YOUTH TOBACCO PRODUCT USE

The following factors are associated with the use of tobacco products among youth:

- Social and physical environments
  - The way mass media show tobacco product use as a normal activity can make young people want to try these products.
  - Youth are more likely to use tobacco products if they see people their age using these products.
  - High school athletes are more likely to use smokeless tobacco than those of the same age who are not athletes.
  - Young people may be more likely to use tobacco products if a parent uses these products.
- Biological and genetic factors
  - There is evidence that youth may be sensitive to nicotine and that teens can feel dependent on nicotine sooner than adults.
  - Genetic factors may make quitting smoking harder for young people.
  - Smoking during pregnancy may increase the likelihood that the child will smoke cigarettes regularly in the future.
- Mental health
  - There is a strong relationship between youth smoking and depression, anxiety, and stress.
- Personal views
  - When young people expect positive things from smoking, such as coping with stress better or losing weight, they are more likely to smoke.

Other influences that affect youth tobacco use include:

- lower socioeconomic status, including lower income or education
- not knowing how to say no to tobacco product use
- lack of support or involvement from parents
- accessibility, availability, and price of tobacco products

- doing poorly in school
- low self-image or self-esteem
- seeing tobacco product advertising in stores, on television, on the Internet, in movies, or in magazines and newspapers

REDUCING YOUTH TOBACCO PRODUCT USE

National, state, and local program activities have been shown to reduce and prevent youth tobacco product use when implemented together. These activities include the following:

- higher costs for tobacco products (e.g., through increased taxes)
- prohibiting smoking in indoor areas of workplaces and public places
- raising the minimum age of sale for tobacco products to 21 years
- television and radio commercials, posters, and other media messages aimed at kids and teens to counter tobacco product ads
- community programs and school and college policies that encourage tobacco-free places and lifestyles
- community programs that lower tobacco advertising and promotions and help make tobacco products less easily available

Some social and environmental factors are related to lower smoking levels among youth. Among these are:

- being part of a religious group or tradition
- racial or ethnic pride and strong racial identity
- higher academic achievement

It is important to keep working to prevent and reduce the use of all forms of tobacco products among youth.[1]

[1] "Youth and Tobacco Use," Centers for Disease Control and Prevention (CDC), November 2, 2023. Available online. URL: www.cdc.gov/tobacco/data_statistics/fact_sheets/youth_data/tobacco_use/index.htm. Accessed April 10, 2024.

Section 12.2 | **Adult Tobacco Use**

SMOKING AND CIGARETTES

Smoking leads to disease and disability and harms nearly every organ of the body. Cigarette smoking remains the leading cause of preventable disease, disability, and death in the United States.

The tobacco industry spends billions of dollars each year on marketing cigarettes. Smoking costs the United States hundreds of billions of dollars annually. However, states do not allocate much of the money they receive from tobacco taxes and lawsuits to prevent smoking and help smokers quit. The Centers for Disease Control and Prevention (CDC) recommends that states spend 12 percent of those funds on tobacco control.

In 2021, 11.5 percent of U.S. adults (an estimated 28.3 million people) smoked cigarettes: 13.1 percent of men and 10.1 percent of women. In 2023, of those youths who ever tried electronic cigarettes (e-cigarettes), approximately half reported using them, indicating that many youths who try e-cigarettes remain e-cigarette users.

Many adult cigarette smokers want to quit smoking.[1]

TRENDS AND MOST RECENT ESTIMATES

By Type of Tobacco Product

Table 12.3 explains the types of tobacco products used by individuals aged 18 and above from 1991 to 2022.

Table 12.3. Percentage of Adults Aged 18 Years and Older Who Reported Tobacco Product Use by Type of Tobacco Product Used, 1991–2022

	Most Recent Estimates (2022)	
Detailed Trend Graphs	**Percent of Adults**	**95% Confidence Interval**
Cigarettes	11.7	11.2–12.2
Smokeless tobacco	2.2	2.0–2.5
Cigars	3.8	3.5–4.1
E-cigarettes	6.6	6.2–7.0

[1] "Fast Facts and Fact Sheets," Centers for Disease Control and Prevention (CDC), November 2, 2023. Available online. URL: www.cdc.gov/tobacco/data_statistics/fact_sheets/fast_facts/index.htm. Accessed April 12, 2024.

Cigarettes, Long-Term Trends (1965+)

Table 12.4 shows the percentage of men and women aged 18 and older who reported smoking cigarettes from 1965 to 2022.

Table 12.4. Percentage of Adults Aged 18 Years and Older Who Reported Cigarette Use by Sex, 1965–2022

	Most Recent Estimates (2022)	
Detailed Trend Graphs	**Percent of Adults**	**95% Confidence Interval**
Both sexes	11.7	11.2–12.2
Male	13.4	12.7–14.2
Female	10.1	9.4–10.7

Cigarettes

BY RACE/ETHNICITY

Table 12.5 shows the number of adults aged 18 and older who reported smoking cigarettes, categorized by their race or ethnicity, from 1991 to 2022.

Table 12.5. Percentage of Adults Aged 18 Years and Older Who Reported Cigarette Use by Race/Ethnicity, 1991–2022

	Most Recent Estimates (2022)	
Detailed Trend Graphs	**Percent of Adults**	**95% Confidence Interval**
All races/ethnicities	11.7	11.2–12.2
Non-Hispanic white	13.0	12.3–13.7
Non-Hispanic Black	14.4	13.0–15.9
Hispanic	8.2	7.2–9.3

BY AGE

Table 12.6 shows the number of adults aged 18 and older who said they smoked cigarettes from 1991 to 2022, sorted by different age groups.

Table 12.6. Percentage of Adults Aged 18 Years and Older Who Reported Cigarette Use by Age, 1991–2022

	Most Recent Estimates (2022)	
Detailed Trend Graphs	**Percent of Adults**	**95% Confidence Interval**
Ages 18–24	4.8	3.7–6.1
Ages 25+	12.7	12.2–13.3

BY POVERTY INCOME LEVEL

Table 12.7 explains the proportion of individuals aged 18 and older who reported smoking cigarettes, categorized according to their income levels by poverty from 1997 to 2022.

Table 12.7. Percentage of Adults Aged 18 Years and Older Who Reported Cigarette Use by Poverty Income Level, 1997–2022

	Most Recent Estimates (2022)	
Detailed Trend Graphs	**Percent of Adults**	**95% Confidence Interval**
<200 percent of federal poverty level	19.6	18.4–20.8
>=200 percent of federal poverty level	8.9	8.4–9.4

BY EDUCATION LEVEL

Table 12.8 shows the percentage of adults aged 25 and older who reported using cigarettes, categorized according to the highest level of education they attained from 1991 to 2022.

Table 12.8. Percentage of Adults Aged 25 Years and Older Who Reported Cigarette Use by Highest Level of Education Obtained, 1991–2022

	Most Recent Estimates (2022)	
Detailed Trend Graphs	**Percent of Adults**	**95% Confidence Interval**
Less than high school	23.1	20.9–25.5
High school	19.2	18.0–20.5
Greater than high school	8.6	8.1–9.2

BY SMOKING FREQUENCY

Table 12.9 shows the proportion of individuals aged 18 and above who have reported their frequency of cigarette smoking from 1991 to 2022. It suggests an analysis of how often adults smoke cigarettes within this time frame.

Table 12.9. Percentage of Adults Aged 18 Years and Older Who Reported Cigarette Use by Smoking Frequency, 1991–2022

	Most Recent Estimates (2022)	
Detailed Trend Graphs	**Percent of Adults**	**95% Confidence Interval**
Nondaily smoking	2.8	2.6–3.1
Daily smoking	8.9	8.5–9.4

Smokeless Tobacco

BY SEX

Table 12.10 shows the statistical representation of the proportion of individuals aged 18 and older who reported using smokeless tobacco categorized by sex from 1993 to 2022. It indicates how the usage of smokeless tobacco has varied among different sexes over the specified time frame.

Table 12.10. Percentage of Adults Aged 18 Years and Older Who Reported Smokeless Tobacco Use by Sex, 1993–2022

	Most Recent Estimates (2022)	
Detailed Trend Graphs	**Percent of Adults**	**95% Confidence Interval**
Both sexes	2.2	2.0–2.5
Male	4.2	3.7–4.7
Female	0.3	0.2–0.4

BY RACE/ETHNICITY

Table 12.11 shows the percentage of smokeless tobacco usage among adults aged 18 and older, segmented by race or ethnicity from 1993 to 2022. It suggests an analysis of how smokeless tobacco consumption patterns vary among different racial and ethnic groups over time.

Table 12.11. Percentage of Adults Aged 18 Years and Older Who Reported Smokeless Tobacco Use by Race/Ethnicity, 1993–2022

	Most Recent Estimates (2022)	
Detailed Trend Graphs	**Percent of Adults**	**95% Confidence Interval**
All races/ethnicities	2.2	2.0–2.5
Non-Hispanic white	3.2	2.8–3.6
Non-Hispanic Black	0.6	0.4–1.0
Hispanic	0.5	0.3–0.8

BY AGE

Table 12.12 explains the percentage of adults aged 18 and older who reported using smokeless tobacco from 1993 to 2022 by different age groups. It indicates how the prevalence of smokeless tobacco use has changed among various age demographics over the specified period.

Table 12.12. Percentage of Adults Aged 18 Years and Older Who Reported Smokeless Tobacco Use by Age, 1993–2022

	Most Recent Estimates (2022)	
Detailed Trend Graphs	**Percent of Adults**	**95% Confidence Interval**
Ages 18–24	1.6	1.0–2.4
Ages 25+	2.3	2.0–2.6

BY POVERTY INCOME LEVEL

Table 12.13 shows the percentage of adults aged 18 and older who reported using smokeless tobacco categorized according to their income level relative to the poverty line from 2000 to 2022.

It suggests an analysis of how smokeless tobacco use patterns may vary among different socioeconomic groups defined by their income levels.

Table 12.13. Percentage of Adults Aged 18 Years and Older Who Reported Smokeless Tobacco Use by Poverty Income Level, 2000–2022

Detailed Trend Graphs	Most Recent Estimates (2022)	
	Percent of Adults	**95% Confidence Interval**
<200 percent of federal poverty level	1.9	1.5–2.3
>=200 percent of federal poverty level	2.3	2.0–2.7

BY EDUCATION LEVEL

Table 12.14 explains the percentage of adults aged 25 and older who reported using smokeless tobacco, categorized based on the highest level of education they attained from 1993 to 2022. It suggests an analysis of how smokeless tobacco use correlates with educational achievement over time.

Table 12.14. Percentage of Adults Aged 25 Years and Older Who Reported Smokeless Tobacco Use by Highest Level of Education Obtained, 1993–2022

Detailed Trend Graphs	Most Recent Estimates (2022)	
	Percent of Adults	**95% Confidence Interval**
Less than high school	2.2	1.6–3.1
High school	3.4	2.8–4.0
Greater than high school	1.9	1.6–2.2

Cigars

BY SEX

Table 12.15 shows the proportion of individuals aged 18 and older who reported cigar usage, divided by gender, from 1998 to 2022.

Table 12.15. Percentage of Adults Aged 18 Years and Older Who Reported Cigar Use by Sex, 1998–2022

	Most Recent Estimates (2022)	
Detailed Trend Graphs	**Percent of Adults**	**95% Confidence Interval**
Both sexes	3.8	3.5–4.1
Male	6.5	6.0–7.1
Female	1.2	1.0–1.5

BY RACE/ETHNICITY

Table 12.16 shows the percentage of adults aged 18 and older who reported using cigars, organized by race/ethnicity, from 1998 to 2022.

Table 12.16. Percentage of Adults Aged 18 Years and Older Who Reported Cigar Use by Race/Ethnicity, 1998–2022

	Most Recent Estimates (2022)	
Detailed Trend Graphs	**Percent of Adults**	**95% Confidence Interval**
All races/ethnicities	3.8	3.5–4.1
Non-Hispanic white	4.1	3.7–4.5
Non-Hispanic Black	5.8	4.7–7.1
Hispanic	2.5	2.0–3.2

BY AGE

Table 12.17 provides the proportion of adults aged 18 and older who have reported using cigars according to different age groups from 1998 to 2022. It provides how cigar use varies across different age demographics over the specified period.

Table 12.17. Percentage of Adults Aged 18 Years and Older Who Reported Cigar Use by Age, 1998–2022

	Most Recent Estimates (2022)	
Detailed Trend Graphs	**Percent of Adults**	**95% Confidence Interval**
Ages 18–24	3.3	2.4–4.5
Ages 25+	3.9	3.6–4.2

BY POVERTY INCOME LEVEL

Table 12.18 explains the percentage of adults aged 18 and older who reported using cigars. The data in this table are organized based on poverty income levels, which categorize individuals into different socioeconomic groups based on their income relative to the poverty line.

Table 12.18. Percentage of Adults Aged 18 Years and Older Who Reported Cigar Use by Poverty Income Level, 1998–2022

	Most Recent Estimates (2022)	
Detailed Trend Graphs	**Percent of Adults**	**95% Confidence Interval**
<200 percent of federal poverty level	4.0	3.4–4.6
>=200 percent of federal poverty level	3.8	3.4–4.1

BY EDUCATION LEVEL

Table 12.19 shows the percentage of adults aged 25 and older who reported using cigars, categorized by their highest level of education from 1998 to 2022. It explains how cigar use varies among adults based on their educational attainment over this period of time.

Table 12.19. Percentage of Adults Aged 25 Years and Older Who Reported Cigar Use by Highest Level of Education Obtained, 1998–2022

	Most Recent Estimates (2022)	
Detailed Trend Graphs	**Percent of Adults**	**95% Confidence Interval**
Less than high school	2.6	1.8–3.7
High school	4.2	3.6–4.9
Greater than high school	4.0	3.6–4.4

E-cigarettes

BY SEX

Table 12.20 provides the percentage of adults aged 18 and older who reported using e-cigarettes, categorized by sex, from 2014 to 2022. It likely presents data showing the prevalence of e-cigarette use among adults over this period, broken down by gender.

Table 12.20. Percentage of Adults Aged 18 Years and Older Who Reported E-cigarette Use by Sex, 2014–2022

	Most Recent Estimates (2022)	
Detailed Trend Graphs	**Percent of Adults**	**95% Confidence Interval**
Both sexes	6.6	6.2–7.0
Male	7.4	6.8–8.1
Female	5.8	5.2–6.4

BY RACE/ETHNICITY

Table 12.21 shows the percentage of adults aged 18 years and older who reported using e-cigarettes, categorized by race or ethnicity. The data spans from the year 2014 to 2022, providing insights into the prevalence of e-cigarette use across different demographic groups over this period.

Table 12.21. Percentage of Adults Aged 18 Years and Older Who Reported E-cigarette Use by Race/Ethnicity, 2014–2022

	Most Recent Estimates (2022)	
Detailed Trend Graphs	**Percent of Adults**	**95% Confidence Interval**
All races/ethnicities	6.6	6.2–7.0
Non-Hispanic white	8.3	7.7–9.0
Non-Hispanic Black	4.8	3.9–5.9
Hispanic	3.7	3.1–4.4

BY AGE

Table 12.22 explains the percentage of adults aged 18 and older who reported using e-cigarettes by age group from 2014 to 2022. It indicates the prevalence of e-cigarette use among different age demographics over a nine-year period.

Table 12.22. Percentage of Adults Aged 18 Years and Older Who Reported E-cigarette Use by Age, 2014–2022

	Most Recent Estimates (2022)	
Detailed Trend Graphs	**Percent of Adults**	**95% Confidence Interval**
Ages 18–24	15.2	13.3–17.4
Ages 25+	5.3	4.9–5.7

BY SEX AND AGE

Table 12.23 presents the percentage of adults aged 18 and older who reported using e-cigarettes. The data is categorized by sex and age groups from 2014 to 2022, showing the trend of e-cigarette use over these years.[2]

Table 12.23. Percentage of Adults Aged 18 Years and Older Who Reported E-cigarette Use by Sex and Age, 2014–2022

	Most Recent Estimates (2022)	
Detailed Trend Graphs	**Percent of Adults**	**95% Confidence Interval**
Males, Ages 18–24	16.8	14.1–19.8
Males, Ages 25+	6.0	5.5–6.6
Females, Ages 18–24	13.7	11.1–16.8
Females, Ages 25+	4.6	4.1–5.1

[2] "Adult Tobacco Use," National Cancer Institute (NCI), March 2024. Available online. URL: https://progressreport.cancer.gov/prevention/adult_smoking#field_most_recent_estimates. Accessed April 23, 2024.

Section 12.3 | Smoking Prevalence among Sexual Minority and Transgender Adults

Smoking prevalence is higher among sexual minority adults than straight adults. In 2020, 16.1 percent of lesbian, gay, or bisexual adults smoked cigarettes, compared to 12.3 percent of heterosexual or straight adults. The use of any commercial tobacco* product was also higher among lesbian, gay, or bisexual adults than among heterosexual or straight adults (25.1 percent versus 18.8 percent).

Transgender adults are more likely to use a commercial tobacco product than cisgender adults. The prevalence of electronic cigarette (e-cigarette) use among transgender adults is more than four times that of cisgender adults (21.3 percent versus 5.0 percent). In 2021, 17.4 percent of gay, lesbian, or bisexual high school students currently used any tobacco product, compared to 11.4 percent of heterosexual high school students. Among middle school students, current use of any tobacco product was three times higher for gay, lesbian, or bisexual youth than for heterosexual youth. About one in five lesbian, gay, or bisexual middle and high school students used e-cigarettes in 2020, compared to about one in eight heterosexual students.

Lesbian, gay, and bisexual adults have more risk factors for cardiovascular disease, such as high blood pressure (HBP), than straight adults. Cigarette smoking can cause cardiovascular disease. Cigarette smoking is the leading cause of lung cancer in all Americans and is linked to at least 11 other types of cancer. Given that an estimated 45,000 lesbian, gay, bisexual, transgender, queer or questioning, or another diverse gender identity (LGBTQ+) people die from cancer each year, it is important to understand the causes of cancer in this population.

Gay, bisexual, and other men who have sex with men (MSM) are the population group most affected by human immunodeficiency virus (HIV) in the United States, with MSM accounting for 69 percent of all new HIV diagnoses. People living with HIV,

* *"Commercial tobacco" refers to harmful products made and sold by tobacco companies. It does not include "traditional tobacco" used by Indigenous groups for religious or ceremonial purposes.*

including those who have access to freely available and well-organized HIV treatment, now lose more years of life from smoking than from HIV.[1]

THE TOBACCO INDUSTRY TARGETS THE LGBTQ+ COMMUNITY WITH MARKETING AND ADVERTISING

Marketing plays a significant role in whether people try or use commercial tobacco products. Being exposed to commercial tobacco ads makes smoking appear more appealing and increases the chance that someone will try smoking for the first time or start using commercial tobacco products regularly.

Tobacco companies spend billions of dollars each year to aggressively market their products. They also target specific populations, including the LGBTQ+ community, and flood them with commercial tobacco advertising.

- **Donations and sponsorships.** In the early 1990s, tobacco companies were among the first large corporations to advertise in magazines and newspapers targeted at LGBTQ+ readers, sponsor Pride parades, and give donations to organizations serving LGBTQ+ people. Tobacco companies stated in internal documents that these sponsorships and ads were marketing tactics designed to attract LGBTQ+ people to their products. In the 1990s, they gave one LGBTQ+ marketing strategy the code name "Project SCUM (Sub-Culture Urban Marketing)." Tobacco companies still advertise at festivals and other community events held by and for LGBTQ+ people and donate to local and national groups serving LGBTQ+ people and people living with HIV.
- **Targeted advertising.** Tobacco companies advertise heavily in publications with gay and lesbian readership, often using images that show LGBTQ+ people using tobacco as a "normal" part of life.

[1] "LGBTQ+ People Experience a Health Burden from Commercial Tobacco," Centers for Disease Control and Prevention (CDC), May 15, 2024. Available online. URL: www.cdc.gov/tobacco-health-equity/collection/lgbtq-health-burden.html. Accessed July 22, 2024.

- **Nightlife marketing.** Bars and clubs have traditionally been one of the few spaces where LGBTQ+ people have felt safe to meet and socialize openly. Tobacco companies work to promote their brands in these spaces and sponsor nightclub after-parties in bars and clubs.
- **Marketing flavored tobacco products to LGBTQ+ people using symbolism.** Adding flavors (such as menthol) to commercial tobacco products can mask the harshness of tobacco, promote youth initiation, lead to the establishment of product use, and contribute to lifelong tobacco use. Ads for flavored tobacco products have used LGBTQ+ symbolism, including phrases like "Take pride in your flavor" or images of colored packages arranged in a rainbow pattern. Tobacco companies have also heavily marketed menthol cigarettes to LGBTQ+ people. This helps explain why about 36 percent of LGBTQ+ people who smoke use menthol cigarettes compared to 29 percent of straight people who smoke.

Public health strategies can help reduce the pressure to buy that comes with heavy advertising and discounts. To help protect LGBTQ+ people from tobacco price promotions and discourage tobacco product use, states and communities could consider increasing prices and prohibiting price discounts, prohibiting the sale of flavored tobacco products, and either allowing fewer stores in a neighborhood to sell commercial tobacco products or prohibiting tobacco product sales altogether.

Other steps that states and communities can take include the following:

- making all workplaces smokefree—with no exceptions
- covering many workplaces by smoke-free laws—but gaps in smoke-free protections often leave out bars and nightclubs
- ensuring that in places without comprehensive smoke-free laws, bartenders and servers in LGBTQ+ nightclubs are not exposed to secondhand smoke

STRESS AND COMMERCIAL TOBACCO USE

When people face many forms of stress—such as financial problems, discrimination, or unsafe neighborhoods—they can be more likely to smoke. Most LGBTQ+ people report experiencing some form of harassment or discrimination because of their sexual orientation or gender identity. More than half have had slurs used against them, and 57 percent report that they or a close friend have been threatened with violence.

The link between discrimination, stress, and commercial tobacco use helps explain why:

- gay college students are more likely to smoke when they have to hide their orientation
- transgender people who have faced discrimination that does not respect their gender identity—such as having to use identifications (IDs) with the wrong gender—are more likely to smoke than transgender people who are supported in their gender identity
- LGBTQ+ youth who attend schools with LGBT-friendly policies and student groups are less likely to begin smoking

When people experience severe or long-lasting stress, their bodies respond by raising stress hormones and keeping them raised. When this continues for a long time, they may develop health problems such as HBP or a faster heart rate. Smoking cigarettes also leads to disease and disability and harms nearly every organ in the body.[2]

[2] "Unfair and Unjust Practices Harm LGBTQ+ People and Drive Health Disparities," Centers for Disease Control and Prevention (CDC), May 15, 202. Available online. URL: www.cdc.gov/tobacco-health-equity/collection/lgbtq-unfair-and-unjust.html. Accessed July 22, 2024.

Section 12.4 | Smoking Patterns among Racial and Ethnic Groups in the United States

Smoking patterns in the United States exhibit significant diversity among different racial and ethnic groups. Individuals of Asian and Hispanic/Latinx descent demonstrate the lowest prevalence of smoking compared to those of other backgrounds. The following explores the smoking habits and associated health risks among African-American, American Indian/Alaska Native, Asian-American, and Hispanic/Latinx populations.

AFRICAN-AMERICAN PEOPLE

Smoking cigarettes puts you at risk for heart disease, cancer, and stroke, which are among the leading causes of death for African-American adults in the United States. About one in eight (11.7 percent) non-Hispanic Black adults in the United States smokes cigarettes. Several factors connect commercial tobacco with higher levels of disease, disability, and death in different population groups.[1]

AMERICAN INDIAN AND ALASKA NATIVE PEOPLE

Cigarette smoking is more common among American Indian and Alaska Native (AI/AN) people than almost any other racial or ethnic group in the United States. In 2020, more than one in four (27.1 percent) American Indian/Alaska Native adults smoked cigarettes. Several factors connect commercial tobacco with higher levels of disease, disability, and death in different population groups.

Smoking increases the chances of:

- losing members from your tribal community to smoking-related illnesses
- losing elders to smoking-related diseases or exposure to secondhand smoke before they can pass down tribal customs and traditions

[1] "African American People," Centers for Disease Control and Prevention (CDC), February 5, 2024. Available online. URL: www.cdc.gov/tobacco/campaign/tips/groups/african-american.html. Accessed April 12, 2024.

If you are a member of an American Indian or Alaska Native community, you likely know someone with health problems from cigarette smoking—possibly a family member with a cough who struggles to breathe or a friend with lung cancer. Smoking cigarettes while you are pregnant increases the risk of pregnancy complications. These health problems may be a special risk in AI/AN communities, where smoking during pregnancy is more common than among other ethnic groups.

If you smoke during pregnancy, you may give birth to a premature baby or a baby who weighs less than 5½ pounds. Sudden infant death syndrome (SIDS; known as "crib death") is another danger for babies of moms who smoke during pregnancy. Babies and children who are exposed to cigarette smoke can continue to have health problems, including bronchitis, pneumonia, and ear infections. You can help protect future generations by keeping children away from cigarette smoke.[2]

ASIAN-AMERICAN PEOPLE

Smoking raises your risk for cancer, heart disease, and stroke, which are among the leading causes of death for people who are Asian American. About 1 in every 20 (5.4 percent) non-Hispanic Asian adults smokes cigarettes. Among Asian-American adults, cigarette smoking is more common in men than in women. Several factors connect commercial tobacco with higher levels of disease, disability, and death in different population groups.[3]

HISPANIC AND LATINX PEOPLE

Cigarette smoking increases your risk for heart disease and cancer, which are the leading causes of death for Hispanic and Latinx people in the United States. About 1 in 13 (7.7 percent) Hispanic or Latinx adults in the United States smoke cigarettes. Among Hispanic and

[2] "American Indian and Alaska Native People," Centers for Disease Control and Prevention (CDC), February 5, 2024. Available online. URL: www.cdc.gov/tobacco/campaign/tips/groups/american-indian-alaska-native.html. Accessed April 12, 2024.

[3] "Asian American People," Centers for Disease Control and Prevention (CDC), February 5, 2024. Available online. URL: www.cdc.gov/tobacco/campaign/tips/groups/asian-american.html. Accessed April 12, 2024.

Latinx people, cigarette smoking is more common in men than in women. Several factors connect commercial tobacco with higher levels of disease, disability, and death in different population groups.

Understanding the smoking patterns and associated health risks among different racial and ethnic groups is crucial for developing targeted public health interventions. Addressing these disparities can help reduce the burden of smoking-related diseases and improve overall health outcomes for these diverse populations.[4]

Section 12.5 | Promoting Smoking Cessation among People with Disabilities

In the United States, one in four adults (an estimated 61.4 million) have a functional disability. These individuals report having serious difficulty with hearing, vision, cognition, mobility, self-care, and/or independent living.

Adults with disabilities are more likely to smoke cigarettes than those without disabilities. About one in five (18.5%) U.S. adults with disabilities smoke cigarettes compared to 10.9 percent of adults without disabilities. Smoking increases the risk of smoking-related illness and death and is the leading preventable cause of disease and death.

Quitting smoking improves quality of life (QOL), reduces the risk of many smoking-related diseases, and can add up to 10 years to life expectancy. Treatments to help people quit include counseling and quit-smoking medications.[1]

PUBLIC HEALTH PROGRAMS AND CAMPAIGNS

Access to proven smoking cessation treatments and services, along with public information campaigns, can significantly reduce

[4] "Hispanic and Latino People," Centers for Disease Control and Prevention (CDC), February 5, 2024. Available online. URL: www.cdc.gov/tobacco/campaign/tips/groups/hispanic-latino.html. Accessed April 12, 2024.

[1] "People with Disabilities," Centers for Disease Control and Prevention (CDC), February 5, 2024. Available online. URL: www.cdc.gov/tobacco/campaign/tips/groups/disabilities.html. Accessed April 12, 2024.

health-care costs and save lives, including those of people with disabilities. Evidence shows that comprehensive tobacco control programs can reduce smoking rates, tobacco-related deaths, and diseases caused by smoking.

To reduce and prevent smoking among people with disabilities, public health programs can:

- include disability in public health surveys and research activities
- update existing health promotion campaigns or programs with targeted smoking cessation messages for people with disabilities
- include people with disabilities in health promotion activities

THE CENTERS FOR DISEASE CONTROL AND PREVENTION'S EFFORTS

The Centers for Disease Control and Prevention (CDC) funds 19 state Disability and Health Programs (www.cdc.gov/ncbddd/disabilityandhealth/programs.html) that work to improve the health and wellness of people with disabilities by including them in health promotion activities to reduce smoking.

Ohio Disability and Health Program

The Ohio Disability and Health Program (https://nisonger.osu.edu/education-training/ohio-disability-health-program) collaborated with the Ohio Department of Health's Tobacco Use Prevention and Cessation Program (TUPCP) to encourage people with disabilities to use the Ohio Tobacco Quit Line.

Highlights of the program include:

- collaborating with TUPCP to add a disability screener question to the Quitline intake form to track people with disabilities who use the service, allowing the program to track changes in Quitline use by people with disabilities over time
- creating a mass media campaign to raise awareness of the Quitline among people with disabilities, with focus groups gathering feedback from the disability

community to develop effective marketing materials; during the three-month campaign, the proportion of callers with a disability increased by 25 percent
- engaging in a Tobacco Cessation Community of Practice with TUPCP and National Jewish Health (provider of the Ohio Tobacco Quitline), resulting in disability sensitivity training for Tobacco Quitline counselors

Michigan Department of Health and Human Services

Members of the Disability and Health and Tobacco units at Michigan Department of Health and Human Services (MDHHS) are working together to promote the Michigan Tobacco Quitline among people with disabilities.

Highlights of the program include:

- training vocational service specialists at Peckham Industries, the largest vocational rehabilitation agency in Lansing, Michigan's capital; since the training, Peckham has changed its policies to automatically refer all employees who wish to quit tobacco to the Michigan Tobacco Quitline
- partnering with a creative advertising class at Michigan State University, where students designed posters and other print materials illustrating the differences in smoking rates for various groups and the importance of accessible smoking cessation resources, raising awareness about access and inclusion among students and providing strong visual messages for promoting the Michigan Tobacco Quitline

New Hampshire Disability and Public Health Program

The New Hampshire Disability and Public Health Program (https://iod.unh.edu/nh-disability-health-program) developed materials for health-care providers to support people with disabilities who want to quit smoking.

Highlights of the program include:

- developing a smoking cessation brochure (https://iod.unh.edu/sites/default/files/media/DPH/tobaccobrochure.pdf)

that offers tips to help people with disabilities quit smoking
- exploring the possibility of including disability identifiers on the state's Quitline intake form
- providing technical assistance and offering training to the New Hampshire Tobacco Prevention and Cessation Program (TPCP) to improve the inclusion and accessibility of the program[2]

Section 12.6 | Smoking and HIV

HOW DOES SMOKING AFFECT YOUR HIV?

In the United States, people living with human immunodeficiency virus (HIV) are twice as likely to smoke as those without the disease. If you have HIV/acquired immunodeficiency syndrome (AIDS) and smoke, you increase your risk of developing both AIDS-related and non-AIDS-related illnesses. Additionally, your HIV medication may not work as well.

You are likely to lose more years of your life to smoking than to HIV itself.

HEALTH PROBLEMS CAUSED BY SMOKING

AIDS-related illnesses include:
- pneumonia
- thrush (a yeast infection in the mouth and throat)
- tuberculosis (TB)
- liver cancer
- HIV-related symptoms such as fatigue, nausea, and body pain

Non-AIDS-related illnesses include:
- lung, head and neck, and other tobacco-related cancers

[2] "Cigarette Smoking among Adults with Disabilities," Centers for Disease Control and Prevention (CDC), November 19, 2020. Available online. URL: www.cdc.gov/ncbddd/disabilityandhealth/smoking-in-adults.html. Accessed April 12, 2024.

- heart disease, including heart attack and stroke
- chronic obstructive pulmonary disease (COPD)[1]

People with HIV who smoke are more likely to have a poorer response to HIV treatment and a shorter lifespan than those who do not smoke. One study found that people with HIV on antiretroviral therapy (ART) with an undetectable viral load who smoke are substantially more likely to die from lung cancer than from HIV itself.

HIV is an independent risk factor for smoking-related cancers, especially for women with HIV. Thus, having HIV increases the risk of smoking-related cancers beyond what is expected from cigarette smoking alone.

Despite declining smoking rates overall in the United States, people with HIV are less likely to quit smoking than the general population.[2]

STATISTICS OF PEOPLE LIVING WITH HIV

Smoking rates among persons living with HIV are much higher than among those without HIV. People living with HIV are also less likely to quit smoking than the general population.

If you have HIV, smoking cigarettes is especially dangerous to your health.

- If you smoke, you are more likely to develop harmful consequences of smoking, such as cancer, heart disease, and stroke, than people without HIV.
- If you smoke, you are more likely to develop HIV-related infections, such as thrush (a mouth infection) and Pneumocystis pneumonia (a lung infection), than someone diagnosed with HIV who does not smoke.
- Among people whose HIV is effectively treated, smoking cigarettes is the main contributor to preventable illness and death.[3]

[1] "HIV and Tobacco Use," U.S. Department of Veterans Affairs (VA), December 15, 2021. Available online. URL: www.mentalhealth.va.gov/quit-tobacco/docs/HIVandTobaccoUse.pdf. Accessed April 12, 2024.

[2] HIV.gov, "Smoking and HIV," U.S. Department of Health and Human Services (HHS), January 26, 2024. Available online. URL: www.hiv.gov/hiv-basics/staying-in-hiv-care/other-related-health-issues/smoking. Accessed April 12, 2024.

[3] "People Living with HIV," Centers for Disease Control and Prevention (CDC), February 5, 2024. Available online. URL: www.cdc.gov/tobacco/campaign/tips/groups/hiv.html. Accessed April 12, 2024.

HEALTH BENEFITS OF QUITTING SMOKING

If you quit smoking, you will decrease your risk of developing:

- heart disease, including heart attack
- cancer
- chronic obstructive pulmonary disease
- pneumonia
- HIV-related symptoms like fatigue[4]

Section 12.7 | Tobacco Use in the Military

SMOKING AND THE MILITARY

High stress levels, peer influence, and military-centric factors such as staying alert for duty may drive tobacco use in the military. Many service members start using tobacco products after they enter military service. Current service members have higher rates of tobacco product use than civilians. In 2018, 18.4 percent of active component service members self-reported current cigarette smoking, and 16 percent self-reported current e-cigarette use. Nearly half, or 47 percent, of current service members who smoked, had tried to quit smoking in the past year. Cigarette smoking is even more common among service members who have recently deployed.[1]

SERVICE MEMBERS AND MILITARY VETERANS

Service members and military veterans have higher rates of tobacco product use than civilians. Cigarette smoking is more common among service members who have been deployed overseas. Smoking increases the risk of lung cancer, heart disease, chronic bronchitis, and many other diseases.

Many service members start using tobacco after they enter military service. During 2010–2015, more than one in five (21.6%) veterans in the United States reported current cigarette smoking.

[4] "HIV and Tobacco Use," U.S. Department of Veterans Affairs (VA), December 15, 2021. Available online. URL: www.mentalhealth.va.gov/quit-tobacco/docs/HIVandTobaccoUse.pdf. Accessed April 12, 2024.

[1] "Be Ready and Determined by Being Tobacco Free," Centers for Disease Control and Prevention (CDC), May 15, 2023. Available online. URL: www.cdc.gov/tobacco/tobacco-features/military.html. Accessed July 22, 2024.

In 2018, 14.6 percent of veterans enrolled for care reported current cigarette smoking.

In addition to adversely affecting their health, the high prevalence of tobacco use among military and veteran personnel also has a significant financial effect. In 2014, the Defense Department spent nearly $1.8 billion on medical and nonmedical costs related to tobacco use. In 2010, the Veterans Health Administration (VHA) spent an estimated $2.7 billion on smoking-related ambulatory care, prescription drugs, hospitalizations, and home health care.

RESOURCES FOR ACTIVE DUTY OR RETIRED SERVICE MEMBERS

Active duty or retired service members, along with their families, may access quitting support through TRICARE coverage and Defense Department programs. If you are in the Reserve or National Guard, check out the following resources:

- The Defense Department's YouCanQuit2 (https://ycq2.org) campaign offers many resources to help people in the U.S. military quit tobacco use.
- Tobacco cessation services (www.tricare.mil/CoveredServices/IsItCovered/TobaccoCessationServices) may be available through TRICARE, including counseling and medications to help you quit tobacco use.[2]

BE READY AND DETERMINED

If you are a service member, you balance demanding job duties to stay mission-ready. The following tips and resources can help you stay tobacco-free:

- **Be ready with a quit-smoking plan**. To get started on your quit journey, visit the Centers for Disease Control and Prevention's (CDC) Guide for Quitting Smoking.
- **Be determined, and do not give up**. It is never too late to quit smoking. Quitting smoking is one of the most important actions you can take to improve your health, regardless of your age or how long you have been smoking.

[2] "Military Service Members and Veterans," Centers for Disease Control and Prevention (CDC), February 5, 2024. Available online. URL: www.cdc.gov/tobacco/campaign/tips/groups/military.html. Accessed April 12, 2024.

Over time, people who quit smoking see many benefits to their health. After you smoke your last cigarette, your body begins a series of positive changes that continue for years. Some health benefits include a drop in heart rate, a decrease in coughing and shortness of breath, and a reduced risk of heart attack, coronary artery disease (CAD), and smoking-related cancer.

Quitting smoking can help you achieve your physical fitness goals. It can also help you be ready and determined for yourself, your family, your friends, and your country.[3]

[3] See footnote [1].

Chapter 13 | Secondhand and Thirdhand Smoke

Chapter Contents

Section 13.1 | **Disparities in Exposure to Secondhand and Thirdhand Smoke**

SECONDHAND AND THIRDHAND SMOKE: PUBLIC HEALTH CONCERNS

Secondhand smoke, or passive or secondary smoke, is a significant public health concern and a driver of smoke-free policies. It increases the risk for many diseases. Exposure to environmental tobacco smoke among nonsmokers increases lung cancer risk by about 20 percent. Secondhand smoke is estimated to cause approximately 53,800 deaths annually in the United States. Exposure to tobacco smoke in the home is also a risk factor for asthma in children.

THIRDHAND SMOKE: EMERGING HEALTH RISKS

Smoking also leaves chemical residue on surfaces where smoking has occurred, which can persist long after the smoke itself has been cleared from the environment. This phenomenon, known as "thirdhand smoke," is increasingly recognized as a potential danger, especially to children. They inhale fumes released by these residues and ingest residues that get on their hands after crawling on floors or touching walls and furniture. Although more research is needed on the risks posed to humans by thirdhand smoke, a study in mice showed that thirdhand smoke exposure has several behavioral and physical health effects, including hyperactivity and adverse effects on the liver and lungs.[1]

THE RIGHT TO SMOKE-FREE AIR

All people deserve a fair and just opportunity to breathe smoke-free air and be as healthy as possible. However, not all populations are equally protected by comprehensive smoke-free laws intended to address exposure to secondhand smoke, making it difficult for everyone to reach their full health potential.

---

[1] "What Are the Effects of Secondhand and Thirdhand Tobacco Smoke?" National Institute on Drug Abuse (NIDA), January 2020. Available online. URL: https://nida.nih.gov/publications/research-reports/tobacco-nicotine-e-cigarettes/what-are-effects-secondhand-thirdhand-tobacco-smoke. Accessed July 22, 2024.

TRENDS AND DISPARITIES IN SECONDHAND SMOKE EXPOSURE

Overview

The proportion of people who do not smoke and are exposed to secondhand smoke has declined in the United States. Despite these gains, disparities in secondhand smoke exposure remain. These disparities exist because of uneven protections and unjust practices. More than one in three people live in a state or community without protection from a comprehensive smoke-free law that prohibits smoking in all workplaces and public places. Many people who live in multiunit housing, like apartment buildings, are exposed to secondhand smoke because smoke travels between units of the same building.

Trends in Secondhand Smoke Exposure in the United States

The percentage of people in the United States who do not smoke and are exposed to secondhand smoke has decreased over the last 60 years. For example, between 1999–2000 and 2011–2012, secondhand smoke exposure among nonsmokers was reduced by half.

Likely reasons for the decline in secondhand smoke exposure include:

- implementation of comprehensive smoke-free laws that prohibit smoking in workplaces, restaurants, and bars
- decreased cigarette smoking prevalence
- increased awareness of the risks of secondhand smoke exposure
- adoption of voluntary smoke-free home rules

Disparity Factors for Secondhand Smoke Exposure

Uneven adoption of smoke-free policies, unfair tobacco industry marketing and advertising practices, and social determinants of health (SDOH) contribute to disparities in secondhand smoke exposure. SDOH refers to the conditions in which people are born, grow, live, work, and age.

Not everyone is protected by comprehensive smoke-free policies that prohibit smoking in all areas. Smoke-free policies protect nonsmokers from secondhand smoke exposure, motivate people who use commercial tobacco to quit, and prevent people from starting to use commercial tobacco. Currently, not everyone in the nation is equally protected by these policies.

As of June 2021, only 3 of the 10 U.S. states with the highest proportion of Black residents have comprehensive smoke-free laws that prohibit smoking in all workplaces and public places. Of the seven states without comprehensive laws, two prevent local communities from adopting comprehensive smoke-free laws. As of July 2022, almost 38 percent of the U.S. population is not protected by comprehensive smoke-free laws at the state or community level. People with lower incomes and less education may be less likely to be covered by comprehensive smoke-free laws. Homes and vehicles remain major sources of secondhand smoke exposure for babies, children, and teens. People living in multiunit housing are more likely to be exposed to secondhand smoke because many buildings lack smoke-free policies. Approximately one in three multiunit housing residents are covered by smoke-free building policies. Secondhand smoke exposure during 2017–2018 was higher among renters (36.6%) than among homeowners (19.2%).

Comprehensive smoke-free laws and policies that prohibit the use of electronic cigarettes (e-cigarettes) can protect nonsmokers from exposure to e-cigarette emissions. The aerosol from e-cigarettes can contain harmful substances.

The tobacco industry has spread misinformation about the dangers of secondhand smoke. A federal court found that tobacco companies deceived the American public about the health effects of secondhand smoke.

POPULATIONS DISPROPORTIONATELY EXPOSED TO SECONDHAND SMOKE

Despite the decline in secondhand smoke exposure, not all populations are equitably protected by smoke-free policies. Some groups remain more likely to be exposed, including:

- children aged 3–11
- non-Hispanic Black people
- people with lower incomes
- people with less education
- people living in rental and multiunit housing

- people living with someone who smokes inside the home
- people working in traditionally "blue-collar" occupations

Children and Adolescents

Almost two of every five children aged 3–11 years, including over half of non-Hispanic Black children, were exposed to secondhand smoke during 2017–2018. An estimated 6.7 million (25.3%) of middle and high school students self-reported secondhand smoke exposure in the home in 2019.

Non-Hispanic Black People

Non-Hispanic Black people (47.2%) had a higher prevalence of secondhand smoke exposure than non-Hispanic Asian people (21.2%), Mexican American people (16.4%), and non-Hispanic white people (22.1%).

People with Lower Incomes

People living below the poverty level (45.0%) have a higher prevalence of secondhand smoke exposure than those with incomes at or above the poverty level (21.4%).

People with Less Education

People aged 25 or older with a high school education (24.3%) or less than high school education (26.4%) have a higher prevalence of secondhand smoke exposure than people with a college diploma or higher (11.1%).

People Living in Rental and Multiunit Housing

An estimated 80 million people—or 25 percent of the U.S. population—live in multiunit housing, such as apartments or condos. People living in rental housing (36.6%) have a higher prevalence of secondhand smoke exposure than homeowners (18.6%). Even when no one in the home smokes, secondhand smoke can drift from other units through hallways, stairwells, and ventilation systems. People living in multiunit housing have higher serum cotinine levels than those living in single-family homes.

People Living with Someone Who Smokes inside the Home

People living with someone who smokes inside the home (87.8%) have a higher prevalence of secondhand smoke exposure than those who do not live with someone who smokes in the home (21.4%).

People Working in Traditionally "Blue-Collar" Occupations

Secondhand smoke exposures in the workplace are more likely among workers in states without comprehensive smoke-free laws. It is also more likely among people working in traditionally "blue-collar" industries, such as construction, industrial machinery, and equipment repair.[2]

Section 13.2 | Health Effects of Secondhand and Thirdhand Smoke

There is no safe level of exposure to secondhand smoke; even brief exposure can cause immediate harm. Health problems caused by secondhand smoke in adults who do not smoke include coronary heart disease, stroke, lung cancer, and adverse reproductive health effects in women, including low birth weight. Secondhand smoke can cause sudden infant death syndrome (SIDS), respiratory infections, ear infections, and asthma attacks in infants and children (see Figure 13.1).

[2] "Trends and Disparities in Secondhand Smoke," Centers for Disease Control and Prevention (CDC), May 15, 2024. Available online. URL: www.cdc.gov/tobacco/secondhand-smoke/disparities.html. Accessed July 22, 2024.

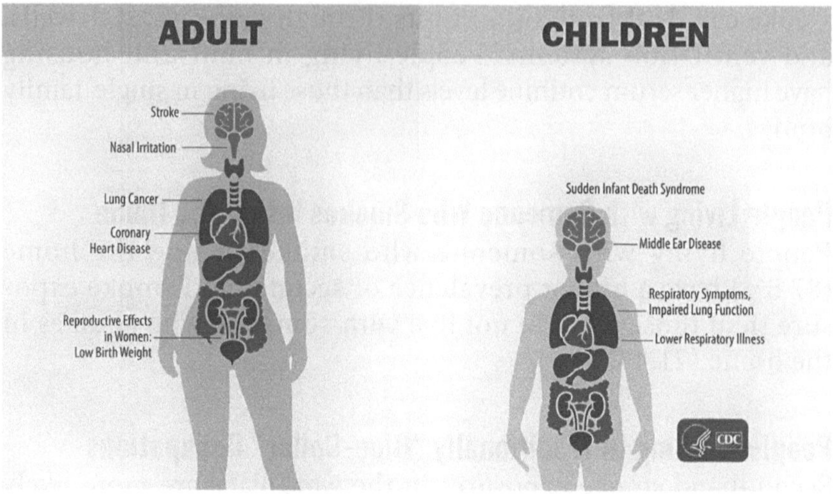

Figure 13.1. Health Effects of Secondhand Smoke on Adults and Children

Centers for Disease Control and Prevention (CDC)

HEALTH PROBLEMS IN ADULTS

Since 1964, approximately 2,500,000 nonsmokers have died from health problems caused by secondhand smoke exposure. In adults who do not smoke, secondhand smoke exposure can cause:

- coronary heart disease
- stroke
- lung cancer
- premature death
- adverse reproductive health effects in women, including low birth weight

Secondhand smoke exposure can produce harmful inflammatory and respiratory effects within 60 minutes of exposure, which can last for at least three hours after exposure.

Heart Disease and Stroke

For adults who do not smoke, exposure to secondhand smoke has immediate harmful effects on the heart and blood vessels and can cause coronary heart disease and stroke. Nearly 34,000 premature deaths from heart disease each year in the United States are attributed to secondhand smoke among nonsmokers. Exposure increases the risk of developing coronary heart disease by 25–30 percent and the risk of stroke by 20–30 percent. Secondhand smoke interferes with the normal functioning of the heart, blood, and vascular systems, increasing the risk of heart attack. Even brief exposure can damage the lining of blood vessels and cause blood platelets to become stickier, increasing the risk of heart attack. People with existing heart disease are at especially high risk and should avoid even brief exposures.

Lung Cancer

Nonsmokers exposed to secondhand smoke increase their risk of developing lung cancer by 20–30 percent. Secondhand smoke causes more than 7,300 lung cancer deaths each year among U.S. adults who do not smoke. Nonsmokers exposed to secondhand smoke inhale many of the same cancer-causing substances and poisons inhaled by smokers. Even brief exposure can damage cells in ways that set the cancer process in motion. The longer the duration and the higher the level of exposure, the greater the risk of developing lung cancer.

Reproductive Health Problems

Women exposed to secondhand smoke during pregnancy are more likely to have newborns with lower birth weights, increasing the risk of health complications.

SUDDEN INFANT DEATH SYNDROME

Infants exposed to secondhand smoke after birth are more likely to die from SIDS than those not exposed. SIDS is the sudden, unexplained, unexpected death of an infant in the first year of life and is the leading cause of death in otherwise healthy infants. Smoking by women during pregnancy increases the risk for SIDS. Chemicals in secondhand smoke affect the brain in ways that interfere with regulating infants' breathing. Infants who die from SIDS have higher concentrations of nicotine in their lungs and higher levels of cotinine, a biological marker for secondhand smoke exposure, than infants who die from other causes.

HEALTH PROBLEMS IN CHILDREN

Children exposed to secondhand smoke are at an increased risk for:

- acute respiratory infections such as pneumonia and bronchitis
- middle ear disease
- more frequent and severe asthma
- respiratory symptoms
- slowed lung growth

Wheezing, coughing, and shortness of breath are more common in children exposed to secondhand smoke. Children whose parents smoke around them have more ear infections and fluid in their ears more often and undergo more operations to insert ear tubes for drainage. Secondhand smoke can trigger asthma attacks in children, and those with asthma who are exposed to secondhand smoke have more severe and frequent asthma attacks. A severe asthma attack can put a child's life in danger.[1]

[1] "Health Problems Caused by Secondhand Smoke," Centers for Disease Control and Prevention (CDC), May 15, 2024. Available online. URL: www.cdc.gov/tobacco/secondhand-smoke/health.html. Accessed July 22, 2024.

Part 2 | Smoking and Tobacco-Related Health Hazards

Chapter 14 | **Health Risks of Smoking**

HEALTH PROBLEMS CAUSED BY SMOKING

Smoking and Death

Cigarette smoking is the leading cause of preventable death in the United States, causing more than 480,000 deaths each year, nearly one in five deaths. Smoking results in more deaths annually than the combined total of human immunodeficiency virus (HIV), illegal drug use, alcohol use, motor vehicle injuries, and firearm-related incidents. More than 10 times as many U.S. citizens have died prematurely from cigarette smoking than in all the wars fought by the United States. Smoking is responsible for about 90 percent of all lung cancer deaths, with more women dying from lung cancer each year than from breast cancer. It also accounts for about 80 percent of all deaths from chronic obstructive pulmonary disease (COPD). Smoking increases the risk of death from all causes in both men and women, and the risk has increased over the last 50 years.

Smoking and Increased Health Risks

Smokers are more likely than nonsmokers to develop heart disease, stroke, and lung cancer. Estimates show that smoking increases the risk:

- for coronary heart disease by two to four times
- for stroke by two to four times
- of men developing lung cancer by 25 times
- of women developing lung cancer by 25.7 times

Smoking leads to diminished overall health, increased absenteeism from work, and higher health-care utilization and costs.

Smoking and Cardiovascular Disease

Smokers are at greater risk for diseases affecting the heart and blood vessels. Smoking causes stroke and coronary heart disease, which are among the leading causes of death in the United States. Even people who smoke fewer than five cigarettes a day can exhibit early signs of cardiovascular disease (CVD). Smoking damages blood vessels, causing them to thicken and narrow, which increases heart rate and blood pressure. Clots can also form. A stroke occurs when a clot blocks the blood flow to part of the brain or when a blood vessel in or around the brain bursts. Blockages caused by smoking can also reduce blood flow to the legs and skin.

Smoking and Respiratory Diseases

Smoking can cause lung disease by damaging the airways and the small air sacs (alveoli) in the lungs. Lung diseases caused by smoking include COPD, which encompasses emphysema and chronic bronchitis. Cigarette smoking is the primary cause of most cases of lung cancer. For individuals with asthma, tobacco smoke can trigger attacks or exacerbate them. Smokers are 12–13 times more likely to die from COPD than nonsmokers.

Smoking and Cancer

Smoking can cause cancer almost anywhere in the body, including the:

- bladder
- blood (acute myeloid leukemia (AML))
- cervix
- colon and rectum (colorectal)
- esophagus
- kidney and ureter
- larynx
- liver
- oropharynx (parts of the throat, tongue, soft palate, and tonsils)
- pancreas
- stomach
- trachea, bronchus, and lung

Smoking increases the risk of dying from cancer and other diseases in cancer patients and survivors. If nobody smoked, one in every three cancer deaths in the United States would not occur.

Smoking and Other Health Risks

Smoking harms nearly every organ of the body and affects overall health. It can make it harder for a woman to become pregnant and can affect her baby's health before and after birth. Risks include preterm delivery, stillbirth, low birth weight, sudden infant death syndrome (SIDS), ectopic pregnancy, and orofacial clefts in infants. Smoking can also affect men's sperm, reducing fertility and increasing risks of birth defects and miscarriage.

Smoking affects bone health, with women past childbearing years who smoke having weaker bones and a greater risk of broken bones. It also affects dental health, increasing the risk of tooth loss. Smoking can increase the risk of cataracts and age-related macular degeneration (AMD), which affects central vision.

Smoking is a cause of type 2 diabetes mellitus (T2DM) and can complicate its control, with a 30–40 percent higher risk for active smokers. It also causes general adverse effects on the body, including inflammation and decreased immune function, and is a cause of rheumatoid arthritis (RA).

QUITTING AND REDUCED RISKS

Quitting smoking is one of the most important actions people can take to improve their health, regardless of age or smoking history.[1]

IS IT HARMFUL TO SMOKE JUST A FEW CIGARETTES A DAY?

There is no safe level of smoking. Even smoking just one cigarette per day over a lifetime can cause smoking-related cancers (lung, bladder, and pancreas) and premature death.[2]

---

[1] "Health Effects of Cigarette Smoking," Centers for Disease Control and Prevention (CDC), October 29, 2021. Available online. URL: www.cdc.gov/tobacco/data_statistics/fact_sheets/health_effects/effects_cig_smoking/index.htm. Accessed April 17, 2024.

[2] "Harms of Cigarette Smoking and Health Benefits of Quitting," National Cancer Institute (NCI), December 19, 2017. Available online. URL: www.cancer.gov/about-cancer/causes-prevention/risk/tobacco/cessation-fact-sheet. Accessed April 17, 2024.

Chapter 15 | Smoking and Cancer

Chapter Contents

CANCER OVERVIEW

Cancer refers to diseases in which cells divide uncontrollably and can invade or spread to other parts of the body. Cancer cells spread through the blood and lymph systems, which help the body eliminate toxins.

There are more than 100 different types of cancer. Most cancers are named after the organ or type of cell in which they start. For example, lung cancer begins in the lung, and laryngeal cancer begins in the larynx (voice box).[1]

TOBACCO USE CAUSES MANY CANCERS

Tobacco use is the leading preventable cause of cancer and cancer deaths. It can cause cancers of the lung, mouth and throat, voice box, esophagus, stomach, kidney, pancreas, liver, bladder, cervix, colon and rectum, and a type of leukemia. Each year, 660,000 people in the United States are diagnosed, and 343,000 people die from cancer related to tobacco use. The Centers for Disease Control and Prevention (CDC) has made progress: more than 1 million tobacco-related cancer deaths have been avoided since 1990 because of comprehensive cancer and tobacco control programs, early detection of cancer, and improvements in cancer treatment. However, not all states or all people have experienced the benefits of these efforts. Greater and longer investments in comprehensive cancer and tobacco control programs can lead to fewer tobacco users and fewer tobacco-related cancers and deaths.[2]

SMOKING AND CANCER

Cigarette smoke contains more than 7,000 chemicals, at least 69 of which can cause cancer. Other chemicals can interfere with the body's ability to fight cancer.

---

[1] "Health Effects of Cigarettes: Cancer," Centers for Disease Control and Prevention (CDC), May 15, 2024. Available online. URL: www.cdc.gov/tobacco/about/cigarettes-and-cancer.html. Accessed July 22, 2024.

[2] "Cancer and Tobacco Use," Centers for Disease Control and Prevention (CDC), November 1, 2016. Available online. URL: www.cdc.gov/vitalsigns/pdf/2016-11-vitalsigns.pdf. Accessed April 17, 2024.

Smoking can also:

- weaken the body's immune system, making it harder to kill cancer cells, allowing them to grow and spread
- damage or change a cell's DNA, causing it to grow out of control and form a tumor

Cigarette smoking causes about one out of every three cancer deaths in the United States. Smoking can cause cancer almost anywhere in the body, including the:

- bladder
- blood (acute myeloid leukemia (AML))
- cervix
- colon and rectum
- esophagus
- kidney and renal pelvis
- larynx (voice box)
- liver
- lung, bronchus, and trachea
- mouth and throat
- pancreas
- stomach

Research suggests that men with prostate cancer who smoke may be more likely to die from prostate cancer than men who do not smoke.

Lung cancer is the leading cause of cancer death in men and women in the United States. Cigarette smoking or secondhand smoke exposure causes nearly 9 out of 10 lung cancer deaths. People who smoke have a greater risk for lung cancer today than they did in 1964, despite smoking fewer cigarettes. Changes in cigarette manufacturing and the chemicals they contain may contribute to this increased risk.

SECONDHAND SMOKE EXPOSURE AND CANCER

Secondhand smoke is smoke from burning tobacco products such as cigarettes, cigars, hookahs, or pipes. Exposure occurs when people breathe in smoke from burning tobacco products or the smoke exhaled by someone smoking.

Secondhand smoke can cause lung cancer in people who have never smoked. In the United States, more than 7,300 people die each year from lung cancer caused by secondhand smoke.

SMOKELESS TOBACCO AND CANCER

Smokeless tobacco, such as chewing tobacco, also causes cancer, including cancer of the:

- esophagus
- mouth and throat
- pancreas

SMOKING AND PEOPLE DIAGNOSED WITH CANCER

Smoking is a serious concern for people with cancer at all stages of the disease and treatment, including after treatment ends. Smoking:

- increases the risk of death, including death from cancer
- increases the risk of developing other smoking-related cancers
- may increase the risk of cancer recurrence (cancer coming back after treatment)
- may result in a poorer response to treatment
- may result in more treatment complications and side effects

QUITTING SMOKING CAN PROTECT PEOPLE FROM CANCER

Quitting smoking is one of the most important actions people can take to improve their health, regardless of age, smoking duration, or amount smoked. Quitting smoking lowers the risk for 12 different cancers, including:

- bladder
- blood (AML)
- cervix
- colon and rectum
- esophagus

- kidney and renal pelvis
- larynx
- liver
- lung, bronchus, and trachea
- mouth and throat
- pancreas
- stomach

The risk of developing cancer decreases over time:
- 5–10 years after quitting, the added risk of cancers of the larynx, oral cavity, and pharynx drops by half
- 10 years after quitting, the risk of cancers of the bladder, esophagus, and kidney decreases
- 10–15 years after quitting, the added risk of lung cancer drops by half
- 20 years after quitting, the risk of cancers of the larynx, oral cavity, pharynx, and pancreas drops to close to that of someone who never smoked
- 20 years after quitting, the added risk of cervical cancer drops by about half

Quitting smoking can also benefit people diagnosed with cancer. Research suggests that people with cancer can reduce their risk of death by quitting smoking. Quitting also improves the prognosis for people with cancer.

CANCER SCREENINGS

Cancer screening involves checking your body for cancer before you have symptoms. Regular screening can help find cancers early when treatment is most effective. Screening is available for three cancers caused by smoking.

Cervical Cancer Screening

Cervical cancer screening with the human papillomavirus (HPV) test and the Pap test can help prevent cervical cancer or find it early. The CDC offers free or low-cost cervical cancer screening nationwide.

Colorectal Cancer Screening

Colorectal cancer screening can find precancerous polyps (abnormal growths) so they can be removed before turning into cancer. Screening tests can also find colorectal cancer early.

Lung Cancer Screening

The U.S. Preventive Services Task Force (USPSTF) recommends lung cancer screening for some adults with a history of heavy smoking. The only recommended screening test for lung cancer is low-dose computed tomography (LDCT).

The USPSTF recommends yearly screening for lung cancer with LDCT for people who:

- have a 20-pack-year or more smoking history
- smoke now or have quit within the past 15 years
- are between 50 and 80 years old

A pack-year is smoking an average of one pack of cigarettes per day for one year. For example, a person could have a 20-pack-year history of smoking one pack a day for 20 years or two packs a day for 10 years.

The USPSTF recommends stopping yearly screening if a person:

- turns 81
- has not smoked for 15 years
- develops a health problem that substantially limits life expectancy
- develops a health problem that makes them unwilling or unable to have surgery if lung cancer is found[3]

PREVENTIVE MEASURES

By Individuals

Everyone can:

- quit using tobacco or never start; quitting at any age will help avoid cancer (Ask a health-care provider for help quitting and call 1-800-QUIT-NOW or visit www.smokefree.gov for free assistance.)

[3] See footnote [1].

- encourage friends, family, and coworkers to quit using tobacco
- teach children and adolescents about the health risks of tobacco use and secondhand smoke exposure
- make their home and vehicle 100 percent tobacco-free and not allow anyone to use tobacco products around children
- learn which cancer screening tests and vaccines are right for them and their family

By Health-Care Providers

Health-care providers can:

- ask all patients whether they use tobacco products, advise those who do not use them not to start, encourage those who do to quit, and provide help with quitting
- help patients understand which cancer screening tests they need and ensure timely screenings
- inform patients that there is no risk-free level of exposure to secondhand smoke and advise them to avoid it
- know which screening and counseling services are reimbursable to their practice

By States and Communities

States and communities can:

- support comprehensive cancer control programs focusing on prevention, education, screening, access to care, support for survivors, and overall health
- fund comprehensive tobacco prevention and control programs at CDC-recommended levels
- make tobacco cessation treatments more available to people who want to quit
- protect nonsmokers from secondhand smoke in all indoor public places and worksites, including all restaurants, bars, and casinos

ACTIONS BY THE FEDERAL GOVERNMENT

The federal government is:

- requiring most insurance plans to cover recommended cancer screenings, vaccinations, and counseling and medications to help people quit tobacco use at no cost to the patient through the Affordable Care Act (ACA)
- funding state tobacco and cancer prevention and control programs to help reduce the number of people who get cancer caused by tobacco use
- funding programs that increase cervical and colorectal cancer screening rates
- regulating the manufacturing, marketing, and distribution of tobacco products
- encouraging smoke-free places that protect nonsmokers from secondhand smoke
- funding and promoting educational campaigns about tobacco use and resources to help people quit

CONTINUING RISK FROM TOBACCO USE

People who use tobacco or are exposed to secondhand smoke are more likely to get and die from cancer. Tobacco smoke has at least 70 carcinogens. Lung and colorectal cancers make up more than half of all cancers linked to tobacco use. Secondhand smoke exposure causes about 7,300 lung cancer deaths among nonsmoking adults each year. About 3 in 10 cancer deaths are caused by cigarette smoking. Lung cancer is the leading cause of cancer death for both men and women.

Quitting tobacco use at any age can reduce the risk of getting or dying from cancer. Getting screened for cancer can lead to fewer cancer cases and deaths from tobacco-related cancers (cervix, colorectal, and lung).

HOW CAN SMOKING-RELATED CANCERS BE PREVENTED?

Quitting smoking lowers the risks of cancers of the lung, mouth, throat, esophagus, and larynx. Within five years of quitting, the chance of developing cancers of the mouth, throat, esophagus, and bladder is cut in half. Ten years after quitting, the risk of dying from lung cancer drops by half. If nobody smoked, one in every three cancer deaths in the United States would not occur.[4]

Section 15.2 | Head and Neck Cancers

Head and neck cancers typically begin in the squamous cells that line the mucosal surfaces of the head and neck, such as those inside the mouth, throat, and voice box. These cancers are called "squamous cell carcinomas" of the head and neck. Less commonly, head and neck cancers can begin in the salivary glands, sinuses, muscles, or nerves.

LOCATIONS WHERE HEAD AND NECK CANCERS FORM

- **Oral cavity**. Includes the lips, the front two-thirds of the tongue, the gums, the lining inside the cheeks and lips, the floor of the mouth under the tongue, the hard palate, and the small area of the gum behind the wisdom teeth.
- **Throat (pharynx)**. A hollow tube about five inches long that starts behind the nose and leads to the esophagus. It has three parts:
  - **Nasopharynx**. The upper part of the pharynx, behind the nose.
  - **Oropharynx**. The middle part of the pharynx, including the soft palate, the base of the tongue, and the tonsils.
  - **Hypopharynx**. The lower part of the pharynx.
- **Voice box (larynx)**. A short passageway formed by cartilage below the pharynx in the neck. It contains the vocal cords and the epiglottis, which prevents food from entering the air passages.

[4] See footnote [2].

- **Paranasal sinuses and nasal cavity.** Small hollow spaces in the bones of the head surrounding the nose and the hollow space inside the nose.
- **Salivary glands.** Located on the floor of the mouth and near the jawbone. They produce saliva and include minor salivary glands throughout the mucous membranes of the mouth and throat.

Cancers of the brain, eye, esophagus, thyroid gland, and skin of the head and neck are not usually classified as head and neck cancers.

If a squamous cell carcinoma of the head and neck spreads, it typically does so locally and/or to the lymph nodes in the neck. Sometimes, cancerous squamous cells can be found in the lymph nodes of the upper neck when there is no evidence of cancer elsewhere in the head and neck, potentially due to the original primary tumor being too small to detect. This condition is known as "metastatic squamous cell carcinoma" with unknown (occult) primary.

SIGNS AND SYMPTOMS OF HEAD AND NECK CANCER

Symptoms of head and neck cancer can include a lump in the neck, a sore in the mouth or throat that does not heal and may be painful, a persistent sore throat, difficulty swallowing, and changes or hoarseness in the voice. Less serious conditions can also cause these symptoms, so it is important to check with a doctor or dentist if they occur.

Specific symptoms based on cancer location include:

- **Oral cavity.** White or red patches on the gums, tongue, or lining of the mouth; growths or swelling of the jaw causing dentures to fit poorly or become uncomfortable; unusual bleeding or pain in the mouth.
- **Throat (pharynx).** Pain when swallowing, persistent neck or throat pain, pain or ringing in the ears, trouble hearing.
- **Voice box (larynx).** Trouble breathing or speaking, pain when swallowing, ear pain.

- **Paranasal sinuses and nasal cavity.** Blocked sinuses that do not clear, chronic sinus infections unresponsive to antibiotics, nosebleeds, frequent headaches, eye swelling or trouble, upper teeth pain, and problems with dentures.
- **Salivary glands.** Swelling under the chin or around the jawbone, facial numbness or muscle paralysis, persistent pain in the face, chin, or neck.

TOBACCO-RELATED CANCERS OF THE HEAD AND NECK

Alcohol and tobacco use, including secondhand smoke and smokeless tobacco, are the two most important risk factors for head and neck cancers, particularly cancers of the oral cavity, hypopharynx, and voice box. People who use both tobacco and alcohol are at a greater risk of developing these cancers than those who use either substance alone. Most head and neck squamous cell carcinomas of the mouth and voice box are caused by tobacco and alcohol use.

REDUCING THE RISK OF HEAD AND NECK CANCERS

Individuals at risk of head and neck cancers, especially tobacco users, should discuss ways to stop using tobacco with their doctor to reduce their risk. Although there is no standard or routine screening test for head and neck cancers, dentists may check the oral cavity for signs of cancer during routine checkups.[1]

Section 15.3 | **Oral Cancer and the Risks of Smokeless Tobacco**

WHAT IS ORAL CANCER?

Oral cancer includes cancers of the mouth and the back of the throat. These cancers develop on the tongue, the tissue lining

[1] "Head and Neck Cancers," Centers for Disease Control and Prevention (CDC), May 25, 2021. Available online. URL: www.cancer.gov/types/head-and-neck/head-neck-fact-sheet#how-can-i-reduce-my-risk-of-developing-head-and-neck-cancers. Accessed April 17, 2024.

the mouth and gums, under the tongue, at the base of the tongue, and in the area of the throat at the back of the mouth. Oral cancer accounts for roughly 3 percent of all cancers diagnosed annually in the United States, with about 54,000 new cases in 2022.

Oral cancer most often occurs in people over the age of 40 and affects more than twice as many men as women. Most cancers in the mouth are related to tobacco use, alcohol consumption, or both, while most throat cancers are caused by the human papillomavirus (HPV). The incidence of HPV-positive oral cancer has risen in recent years.

Signs and Symptoms of Oral Cancer

If you experience any of these symptoms for more than two weeks, see a dentist or doctor:

- a sore, irritation, lump, or thick patch in your mouth, lip, or throat
- a white or red patch in your mouth
- persistent sore throat, a feeling that something is caught in your throat, hoarseness, or loss of your voice
- a lump in the neck
- difficulty chewing, swallowing, or speaking
- difficulty moving your jaw or tongue
- swelling of your jaw causing dentures to fit poorly or become uncomfortable
- pain or bleeding in the mouth
- numbness in your tongue or other areas of your mouth
- ear pain

TOBACCO-RELATED CANCERS OF THE MOUTH

Tobacco use, including cigarette, pipe, cigar, and electronic cigarette smoking, as well as chewing tobacco and snuff, puts you at risk for developing oral cancers.[1]

[1] "Oral Cancer," National Institute of Dental and Craniofacial Research (NIDCR), June 1, 2023. Available online. URL: www.nidcr.nih.gov/health-info/oral-cancer. Accessed April 18, 2024.

WHAT IS SMOKELESS TOBACCO?

Smokeless tobacco is tobacco that is not burned. It is also known as "chewing tobacco," "oral tobacco," "spit or spitting tobacco," "dip," "chew," and "snuff." Most people chew or suck (dip) the tobacco in their mouth and spit out the tobacco juices that build up, although spitless smokeless tobacco has also been developed. Nicotine in the tobacco is absorbed through the lining of the mouth.

People in many regions, including North America, Northern Europe, India, other Asian countries, and parts of Africa, have a long history of using smokeless tobacco products.

Types of Smokeless Tobacco

- **Chewing tobacco**. Available as loose leaves, plugs (bricks), or twists of rope. A piece of tobacco is placed between the cheek and lower lip, typically toward the back of the mouth. It is either chewed or held in place. Saliva is spit or swallowed.
- **Snuff**. Finely cut or powdered tobacco, sold in different scents and flavors, packaged moist or dry. Most American snuff is moist. It is available loose, in dissolvable lozenges or strips, or in small pouches similar to tea bags. A pinch or pouch of moist snuff is placed between the cheek and gums or behind the upper or lower lip. Moist snuff is also known as "snus." Some people inhale dry snuff into the nose.

HARMFUL CHEMICALS IN SMOKELESS TOBACCO

There is no safe form of tobacco. At least 28 chemicals in smokeless tobacco cause cancer. The most harmful chemicals are tobacco-specific nitrosamines, formed during the growing, curing, fermenting, and aging of tobacco. The level of these nitrosamines varies by product and is directly related to cancer risk. Other cancer-causing substances include polonium-210 (a radioactive element in tobacco fertilizer) and polycyclic aromatic hydrocarbons.

HEALTH RISKS OF SMOKELESS TOBACCO

Cancer

Smokeless tobacco causes oral cancer, esophageal cancer, and pancreatic cancer.

Other Diseases

Using smokeless tobacco may also cause heart disease, gum disease, and oral lesions other than cancer, such as leukoplakia (precancerous white patches in the mouth).

Addiction

All tobacco products, including smokeless tobacco, contain nicotine, which is addictive. Users of smokeless tobacco and cigarettes have comparable levels of nicotine in the blood. Nicotine is absorbed through the mouth tissues directly into the blood, where it reaches the brain. Even after the tobacco is removed from the mouth, nicotine continues to be absorbed into the bloodstream and remains in the blood longer than it does for smokers.

The nicotine level in the blood depends on the amount of nicotine in the product, the cut size of the tobacco, the product's pH (acidity or basicity), and other factors. A Centers for Disease Control and Prevention (CDC) study of 40 popular brands of moist snuff showed nicotine levels ranging from 4.4 to 25.0 milligrams per gram of tobacco. Other studies found that moist snuff contained 4.7 to 24.3 milligrams per gram, dry snuff contained 10.5 to 24.8 milligrams per gram, and chewing tobacco contained 3.4 to 39.7 milligrams per gram.

COMPARING RISKS: SMOKELESS TOBACCO VERSUS CIGARETTES

All tobacco products are harmful and cause cancer, so the use of all tobacco products should be strongly discouraged. There is no safe level of tobacco use. People who use any type of tobacco product should be urged to quit. For help with quitting, refer to the National Cancer Institute (NCI) fact sheet "Where To Get Help When You Decide To Quit Smoking" (www.cancer.gov/about-cancer/causes-prevention/risk/tobacco/help-quitting-fact-sheet).

As early as 1986, the advisory committee to the Surgeon General concluded that smokeless tobacco "is not a safe substitute for smoking cigarettes." It can cause cancer, noncancerous oral conditions, and lead to nicotine addiction and dependence. In 2006, a panel of experts convened by the National Institutes of Health (NIH) stated that the "range of risks, including nicotine addiction, from smokeless tobacco products may vary extensively because of differing levels of nicotine, carcinogens, and other toxins in different products."

SHOULD SMOKELESS TOBACCO BE USED TO HELP QUIT SMOKING?

No. There is no scientific evidence that using smokeless tobacco can help a person quit smoking. Because all tobacco products are harmful and cause cancer, their use is strongly discouraged. People who use any type of tobacco product should be urged to quit. For help with quitting, ask your doctor about individual or group counseling, telephone quitlines, or other methods.[2]

Section 15.4 | Lung Cancer

LUNG CANCER BASICS

What It Is

Lung cancer begins in the lungs and can spread to lymph nodes or other organs in the body, such as the brain. Cancer from other organs can also spread to the lungs. When cancer cells spread from one organ to another, they are called "metastases."

Types

Lung cancers are generally grouped into two main types: small cell lung cancer (SCLC) and nonsmall cell lung cancer (NSCLC). NSCLC includes adenocarcinoma and squamous cell carcinoma. These types grow differently and are treated differently. NSCLC is more common than small cell lung cancer.

Symptoms

People with lung cancer can have different symptoms. Some have symptoms related to the lungs, while others whose lung cancer

[2] "Smokeless Tobacco and Cancer," National Cancer Institute (NCI), October 25, 2010. Available online. URL: www.cancer.gov/about-cancer/causes-prevention/risk/tobacco/smokeless-fact-sheet. Accessed April 18, 2024.

has metastasized have symptoms specific to the affected body part. Some people just have general symptoms of not feeling well. Most people with lung cancer do not have symptoms until the cancer is advanced.

Lung cancer symptoms may include:

- coughing that worsens or does not go away
- chest pain
- shortness of breath
- wheezing
- coughing up blood
- feeling very tired all the time
- weight loss with no known cause

Other possible changes include repeated bouts of pneumonia and swollen or enlarged lymph nodes inside the chest between the lungs. These signs and symptoms can also occur with other illnesses. If you experience any of these symptoms, talk to your doctor.

SMOKING

Cigarette smoking is the number one risk factor for lung cancer. In the United States, cigarette smoking is linked to about 80–90 percent of lung cancer deaths. Using other tobacco products, such as cigars or pipes, also increases the risk of lung cancer. Tobacco smoke is a toxic mix of more than 7,000 chemicals, many of which are poisons. At least 70 are known to cause cancer in people or animals.

People who smoke cigarettes are 15–30 times more likely to get lung cancer or die from lung cancer than people who do not smoke. Even smoking a few cigarettes a day or smoking occasionally increases the risk of lung cancer. The more years a person smokes, and the more cigarettes smoked each day, the higher the risk.

People who quit smoking have a lower risk of lung cancer than if they had continued to smoke, but their risk remains higher than that of people who never smoked. Quitting smoking at any age can lower the risk of lung cancer.

Cigarette smoking can cause cancer almost anywhere in the body, including the mouth and throat, esophagus, stomach, colon, rectum, liver, pancreas, voice box (larynx), lung, trachea, bronchus, kidney and renal pelvis, urinary bladder, cervix, and can cause acute myeloid leukemia. Secondhand smoke also causes lung cancer.

SCREENING FOR LUNG CANCER

Screening means testing for a disease when there are no symptoms or history of that disease. Doctors recommend a screening test to find a disease early, when treatment may be more effective.

The only recommended screening test for lung cancer is low-dose computed tomography (LDCT). During an LDCT scan, you lie on a table while an x-ray machine uses a low dose of radiation to make detailed images of your lungs. The scan takes only a few minutes and is not painful.

Who Should Be Screened?

The U.S. Preventive Services Task Force (USPSTF) recommends yearly lung cancer screening with LDCT for people who:

- have a 20-pack-year or more smoking history
- smoke now or have quit within the past 15 years
- are between 50 and 80 years old

A pack-year is smoking an average of one pack of cigarettes per day for one year. For example, a person could have a 20-pack-year history of smoking one pack a day for 20 years or two packs a day for 10 years.

Risks of Screening

Lung cancer screening has at least three risks:

- A false-positive result, which can suggest that a person has lung cancer when no cancer is present. This can lead to unnecessary follow-up tests and surgeries, which may have risks.
- Overdiagnosis, where the screening test finds cases of cancer that may never have caused a problem for the patient, leading to unnecessary treatment.

- Radiation from repeated LDCT tests can cause cancer in otherwise healthy people.

Because of these risks, lung cancer screening is recommended only for adults at high risk for developing the disease due to their smoking history and age. It is not recommended for those who have a health problem that substantially limits life expectancy or their ability or willingness to have lung surgery if needed.

If you are considering screening, discuss it with your doctor, who can refer you to a high-quality screening facility.

REDUCING THE RISK FOR LUNG CANCER

Steps you can take to reduce your risk include:

- **Do not smoke.** Cigarette smoking causes about 80–90 percent of lung cancer deaths in the United States. The most important thing you can do to prevent lung cancer is to not start smoking or to quit if you smoke.
- **Avoid secondhand smoke.** Make your home and car smoke-free.
- **Get your home tested for radon.** The U.S. Environmental Protection Agency (EPA) recommends that all homes be tested for radon.
- **Be careful at work.** Follow health and safety guidelines to avoid carcinogens (things that can cause cancer).

HEALTHY LIVING

It is important to get timely and appropriate care for lung cancer and its symptoms, including pain and treatment side effects. Molecular testing (tumor or biomarker testing) may help make treatment decisions. Genetic testing may also be considered to identify inherited characteristics.

Discuss with your health-care provider how a survivorship care plan can help coordinate your follow-up care and support your physical and emotional health. Taking steps to stay healthy can lower your risk of cancer recurrence.

Some cancer survivors may feel blame or stigma. Talking about your experiences and feelings with a social worker or mental health professional can be helpful. Sharing your story with other cancer survivors or listening to their stories may also provide support.[1]

Section 15.5 | Gastrointestinal Cancers

COLORECTAL CANCER

What Is Colorectal Cancer?

Cancer is a disease in which cells in the body grow out of control. When cancer starts in the colon or rectum, it is called "colorectal cancer." Sometimes, it is referred to simply as "colon cancer." The colon is the large intestine or large bowel, and the rectum is the passageway that connects the colon to the anus.

Abnormal growths called "polyps" can form in the colon or rectum. Over time, some polyps may turn into cancer. Screening tests can find polyps, so they can be removed before turning into cancer. Screening also helps find colorectal cancer at an early stage, when treatment works best.

If you are 45 years old or older, talk to your doctor about screening. If you think you may be at increased risk for colorectal cancer, discuss with your doctor when to begin screening, which test is right for you, and how often to get tested.

Signs and Symptoms of Colorectal Cancer

Colorectal polyps and colorectal cancer do not always cause symptoms, especially at first. You could have polyps or colorectal cancer and not know it, which is why getting screened regularly is crucial.

If you do have symptoms, they may include:

- a change in bowel habits
- blood in or on your stool (bowel movement)

[1] "Lung Cancer Basics," Centers for Disease Control and Prevention (CDC), October 26, 2023. Available online. URL: www.cdc.gov/lung-cancer/about. Accessed July 22, 2024.

- diarrhea, constipation, or feeling that the bowel does not empty completely
- abdominal pain, aches, or cramps that do not go away
- unexplained weight loss

If you experience any of these symptoms, talk to your doctor. These symptoms may be caused by something other than cancer, but the only way to know is to see your doctor.

Causes and Risk Factors of Colorectal Cancer

Your risk of getting colorectal cancer increases as you age. Other risk factors include having:

- inflammatory bowel disease (IBD), such as Crohn's disease or ulcerative colitis
- a personal or family history of colorectal cancer or colorectal polyps
- a genetic syndrome, such as familial adenomatous polyposis (FAP) or hereditary nonpolyposis colorectal cancer (Lynch syndrome)

Lifestyle factors that may contribute to an increased risk of colorectal cancer include:

- lack of regular physical activity
- a diet low in fruits and vegetables
- a low-fiber and high-fat diet, or a diet high in processed meats
- overweight and obesity
- alcohol consumption
- tobacco use

Reducing Risk for Colorectal Cancer

Almost all colorectal cancers begin as precancerous polyps in the colon or rectum. These polyps can be present for years before invasive cancer develops and may not cause any symptoms, especially early on. Colorectal cancer screening can find precancerous polyps, so they can be removed before they turn into cancer, thus preventing colorectal cancer. Screening can also detect colorectal cancer early when treatment is most effective.

Some studies suggest that people may reduce their risk of developing colorectal cancer by:

- increasing physical activity
- maintaining a healthy weight
- eating a diet low in animal fats and high in fruits, vegetables, and whole grains
- limiting alcohol consumption
- avoiding tobacco[1]

ESOPHAGEAL CANCER

What Is Esophageal Cancer?

Esophageal cancer is a disease in which malignant (cancer) cells form in the tissues of the esophagus. The esophagus is the hollow, muscular tube that moves food and liquid from the throat to the stomach. The esophagus wall comprises several layers of tissue, including the mucous membrane, muscle, and connective tissue. Esophageal cancer starts on the inside lining of the esophagus and spreads outward through the other layers as it grows.

The two most common forms of esophageal cancer are named for the type of cells that become malignant:

- **Squamous cell carcinoma**. Cancer that forms in the thin, flat cells lining the inside of the esophagus. This type of cancer is most often found in the upper and middle parts of the esophagus but can occur anywhere along the esophagus. It is also called "epidermoid carcinoma."
- **Adenocarcinoma**. Cancer that begins in glandular cells. These cells in the lining of the esophagus produce and release fluids such as mucus. Adenocarcinomas usually form in the lower part of the esophagus, near the stomach.

---

[1] "Colorectal Cancer Basics," Centers for Disease Control and Prevention (CDC), June 12, 2024. Available online. URL: www.cdc.gov/colorectal-cancer/about. Accessed July 22, 2024.

Signs and Symptoms of Esophageal Cancer

Signs and symptoms of esophageal cancer may include:

- painful or difficult swallowing
- weight loss
- pain behind the breastbone
- hoarseness and cough
- indigestion and heartburn
- a lump under the skin

These symptoms can be caused by esophageal cancer or other conditions. Check with your doctor if you experience any of these symptoms.

What Can You Do to Reduce Your Risk?

Studies have shown that the risk of squamous cell carcinoma of the esophagus is lower in people who do not use tobacco and alcohol. To reduce your risk:

- **Avoid tobacco use**. Refrain from smoking or using other tobacco products.
- **Limit alcohol consumption**. Reduce or eliminate alcohol intake.[2]

LIVER CANCER

What Is Liver Cancer?

Primary liver cancer is a disease in which malignant (cancer) cells form in the tissues of the liver. Cancer that originates in other parts of the body and spreads to the liver is not considered primary liver cancer. The liver is one of the largest organs in the body, located in the upper right side of the abdomen inside the rib cage. Its main functions include:

- producing bile to help digest fats from food
- storing glycogen (sugar), which the body uses for energy

---

[2] "Esophageal Cancer Treatment (PDQ®)–Patient Version," National Cancer Institute (NCI), September 21, 2023. Available online. URL: www.cancer.gov/types/esophageal/patient/esophageal-treatment-pdq. Accessed April 18, 2024.

- filtering harmful substances from the blood, which are then passed from the body in stools and urine

Signs and Symptoms of Liver Cancer

These and other signs and symptoms may be caused by primary liver cancer or by other conditions. Consult your doctor if you experience any of the following:

- a hard lump on the right side just below the rib cage
- discomfort in the upper abdomen on the right side
- a swollen abdomen
- pain near the right shoulder blade or in the back
- jaundice (yellowing of the skin and whites of the eyes)
- easy bruising or bleeding
- unusual tiredness or weakness
- nausea and vomiting
- loss of appetite or feelings of fullness after eating a small meal
- unexplained weight loss
- pale, chalky bowel movements and dark urine
- fever

What Can You Do to Reduce Your Risk of Liver Cancer?

Avoiding tobacco is one of the best ways to reduce your risk of liver cancer. Cigarette smoking has been linked to a higher risk of liver cancer, with the risk increasing with the number of cigarettes smoked per day and the number of years smoked.[3]

Hepatitis C and Tobacco Use

HOW DOES SMOKING AFFECT YOUR LIVER?

The liver processes the food we eat to convert it into energy and acts as a filter for toxic substances that enter our body. When you have hepatitis C, the virus causes your liver to become inflamed and less effective at clearing out toxic substances. Smoking exacerbates

[3] "What Is Liver Cancer?" National Cancer Institute (NCI), May 18, 2022. Available online. URL: www.cancer.gov/types/liver/what-is-liver-cancer. Accessed April 29, 2024.

this issue by adding cancer-causing substances found in tobacco, making your liver work even harder.

WHAT KIND OF PROBLEMS CAN SMOKING CAUSE WITH YOUR HEPATITIS C?

If you have hepatitis C and smoke, you:

- increase your chance of developing liver cancer
- speed up the development of fibrosis, which can progress to cirrhosis
- increase your risk of joint pain, especially in the fingers, back, and knees

These issues are in addition to tobacco-specific problems such as increased risk for certain cancers, chronic obstructive pulmonary disease (COPD), and cardiovascular problems, including stroke.

BENEFITS OF QUITTING SMOKING WITH HEPATITIS C

Quitting smoking can reduce your risk of developing liver cancer and joint pain, and slow down the development of fibrosis. Additionally, quitting will lower your risk of tobacco-related cancers, COPD, and heart disease.[4]

PANCREATIC CANCER

What Is Pancreatic Cancer?

Pancreatic cancer is a type of cancer that forms in the tissues of the pancreas. The pancreas is a gland about six inches long, shaped like a thin pear lying on its side. The wider end of the pancreas is called the "head," the middle section is the "body," and the narrow end is the "tail." The pancreas lies between the stomach and the spine.

The pancreas has two main functions in the body:

- **Digestive**. Produces juices that help break down food into substances the body can use.

[4] "Hepatitis C and Tobacco Use," U.S. Department of Veterans Affairs (VA), July 6, 2018. Available online. URL: www.mentalhealth.va.gov/quit-tobacco/docs/HepatitisCandTobaccoUse_R2.pdf. Accessed April 29, 2024.

- **Endocrine.** Produces hormones, such as insulin and glucagon, that help control blood sugar levels and help the body use and store the energy it gets from food.

Pancreatic cancer can occur in the exocrine cells, which produce digestive juices, or the endocrine cells, which produce hormones. About 95 percent of pancreatic cancers begin in exocrine cells.

Signs and Symptoms of Pancreatic Cancer

Pancreatic cancer may not cause any signs or symptoms early on, making it hard to detect. As the cancer grows, symptoms may include:

- jaundice (yellowing of the skin and whites of the eyes)
- light-colored stools
- dark urine
- pain in the upper or middle abdomen and back
- unexplained weight loss
- loss of appetite
- fatigue

These symptoms can be caused by many conditions other than pancreatic cancer. It is important to check with your doctor if you have any of these symptoms to determine the cause and begin treatment, if needed.

What Can You Do to Reduce Your Risk of Pancreatic Cancer?

Not smoking or quitting smoking lowers the risk of getting cancer and dying from cancer. Scientists believe that cigarette smoking causes about 30 percent of all cancer deaths in the United States. Therefore, avoiding tobacco use is one of the most effective ways to reduce your risk of pancreatic cancer.[5]

---

[5] "Pancreatic Cancer Treatment (PDQ®)–Patient Version," National Cancer Institute (NCI), March 5, 2024. Available online. URL: www.cancer.gov/types/pancreatic/patient/pancreatic-treatment-pdq. Accessed April 29, 2024.

STOMACH CANCER

What Is Stomach Cancer?

Stomach (gastric) cancer is cancer that starts in the cells lining the stomach. The stomach, located on the left side of the upper abdomen, is part of the digestive tract—a series of hollow, muscular organs joined in a long, twisting tube from the mouth to the anus. The digestive tract processes nutrients from foods and helps pass waste material out of the body:

- Food moves from the throat to the stomach through a tube called the "esophagus."
- In the stomach, food is broken down by stomach muscles that mix the food and liquid with digestive juices.
- Partly digested food then passes into the small intestine and subsequently into the large intestine.
- The end of the large intestine, called the "rectum," stores waste from the digested food until it is expelled through the anus during a bowel movement.

Signs and Symptoms of Stomach Cancer

Early-stage stomach cancer usually does not have symptoms, making it hard to detect. Symptoms typically begin after the cancer has spread. When early-stage symptoms do occur, they may include:

- indigestion and stomach discomfort
- a bloated feeling after eating
- mild nausea
- loss of appetite
- heartburn

Symptoms of advanced stomach cancer (cancer that has spread beyond the stomach) may include the early-stage symptoms as well as:

- blood in the stool
- vomiting
- unexplained weight loss
- stomach pain

- jaundice (yellowing of the eyes and skin)
- ascites (buildup of fluid in the abdomen)
- trouble swallowing

These symptoms can be caused by many conditions other than stomach cancer. If you experience any of these symptoms, it is important to check with your doctor. Your doctor will ask when your symptoms started and how often you have been experiencing them. If it is stomach cancer, ignoring symptoms can delay treatment and make it less effective.

Tobacco-Related Stomach Cancer

People who smoke have a higher risk of stomach cancer than nonsmokers. Smoking also makes treatment for *Helicobacter pylori* (*H. pylori*) infection less effective. Smokers who quit smoking lower their risk of developing stomach cancer over time.[6]

What Can You Do to Reduce Your Risk of Stomach Cancer?

Studies have shown that smoking is a key risk factor for gastric cancer. A systematic review and meta-analysis revealed a 60 percent increase in gastric cancer in male smokers and a 20 percent increase in female smokers compared with nonsmokers. Another systematic review addressed the relationship between cigarette smoking and gastric cancer by estimating the association's magnitude for different exposure levels. It provides solid evidence that smoking is the most important behavioral risk factor for gastric cancer. The risk of stomach cancer decreases among former smokers compared with persistent smokers, with the risk decreasing over time since cessation. These observations suggest that cigarette smoking prevention or cessation would result in a decreased risk of gastric cancer.[7]

---

[6] "What Is Stomach Cancer?" National Cancer Institute (NCI), May 31, 2023. Available online. URL: www.cancer.gov/types/stomach. Accessed April 29, 2024.

[7] "Stomach (Gastric) Cancer Prevention (PDQ®)–Health Professional Version," National Cancer Institute (NCI), March 19, 2024. Available online. URL: www.cancer.gov/types/stomach/hp/stomach-prevention-pdq#_138. Accessed April 29, 2024.

Section 15.6 | Gynecological Cancers

WHAT IS CERVICAL CANCER?

Cervical cancer is a disease in which cells in the cervix grow uncontrollably. The cervix connects the vagina (birth canal) to the upper part of the uterus, where a baby grows during pregnancy. Anyone with a cervix is at risk for cervical cancer, which occurs most often in people over age 30. Long-lasting infection with certain types of human papillomavirus (HPV) is the main cause of cervical cancer. HPV is a common virus transmitted through sexual contact. Although at least half of sexually active people will have HPV at some point, few will develop cervical cancer.

Screening tests and the HPV vaccine can help prevent cervical cancer. When found early, cervical cancer is highly treatable, with a good prognosis for long survival and quality of life (QOL).

SIGNS AND SYMPTOMS OF CERVICAL CANCER

Early-stage cervical cancer may not cause signs and symptoms. Advanced cervical cancer may cause abnormal bleeding or discharge from the vagina, such as bleeding after sex. If you experience any of these signs, see your doctor. They may be caused by conditions other than cancer, but only a doctor can determine the cause.[1]

TOBACCO-RELATED CERVICAL CANCER

People who smoke or breathe in secondhand smoke have an increased risk of developing cervical cancer. The risk increases with the amount of smoking and exposure to secondhand smoke. This is because tobacco smoke contains harmful chemicals that can damage the cells of the cervix and weaken the immune system, making it harder for the body to fight off HPV infections, which are the main cause of cervical cancer.[2]

---

[1] "Cervical Cancer Basics," Centers for Disease Control and Prevention (CDC), February 22, 2024. Available online. URL: www.cdc.gov/cervical-cancer/about. Accessed July 22, 2024.

[2] "Cervical Cancer Causes, Risk Factors, and Prevention," National Cancer Institute (NCI), August 18, 2023. Available online. URL: www.cancer.gov/types/cervical/causes-risk-prevention. Accessed April 25, 2024.

SCREENING TESTS

The HPV test and the Pap test can help prevent cervical cancer or detect it early.

- **HPV test.** Looks for the virus that can cause cell changes on the cervix.
- **Pap test (Pap smear).** Looks for precancers—cell changes on the cervix that might become cervical cancer if not treated appropriately.

Both tests can be done in a doctor's office or clinic. During the Pap test, a speculum is used to look inside the vagina and collect cells and mucus from the cervix. These cells are sent to a laboratory for analysis:

- For a Pap test, the cells are checked for abnormalities.
- For an HPV test, the cells are tested for the presence of HPV.

CONDITIONS THAT CAN INCREASE RISK

Almost all cervical cancers are caused by HPV, a common virus passed through sexual contact. HPV types can cause changes on the cervix that can lead to cervical cancer over time, while other types can cause genital or skin warts. HPV often has no symptoms, so many people do not know they have it. Although HPV usually goes away on its own, it can cause cervical cancer if it persists. Other factors that increase cervical cancer risk include:

- having HIV or another condition that weakens the immune system
- tobacco smoking

HUMAN PAPILLOMAVIRUS VACCINE

The HPV vaccine protects against the types of HPV that most often cause cervical, vaginal, and vulvar cancers.

- **Recommended age.** The vaccine is recommended for preteens aged 11–12 years but can be given starting at age 9.
- **Age range.** HPV vaccination is recommended for everyone through age 26 if not already vaccinated. It is

not generally recommended for people older than 26, but some adults aged 27 through 45 may choose to get vaccinated after discussing their risk with a doctor.
- **Dosage.** A two-dose schedule is recommended if vaccination starts before age 15, with doses given 6–12 months apart. For those starting after their 15th birthday, a three-shot series is required.

The HPV vaccine prevents new HPV infections but does not treat existing infections or diseases. It works best when given before exposure to HPV. Regular cervical cancer screenings are necessary even for those who have received the HPV vaccine.[3]

OVARIAN, FALLOPIAN TUBE, AND PRIMARY PERITONEAL CANCERS

What They Are

The ovarian, fallopian tube, and primary peritoneal cancers are diseases in which malignant (cancer) cells form in the ovaries, fallopian tubes, or peritoneum.

- **Ovaries.** A pair of organs in the female reproductive system, located in the pelvis, one on each side of the uterus. They are about the size and shape of an almond and are responsible for making eggs and female hormones.
- **Fallopian tubes.** A pair of long, slender tubes on each side of the uterus. Eggs pass from the ovaries, through the fallopian tubes, to the uterus. Cancer can begin at the end of the fallopian tube near the ovary and spread to the ovary.
- **Peritoneum.** The tissue lining the abdominal wall and covering the organs in the abdomen. Primary peritoneal cancer forms in the peritoneum and has not spread there from another part of the body. It can spread to the ovary.

Ovarian cancer is the leading cause of death from cancer of the female reproductive system. It is most common in postmenopausal

[3] See footnote [1].

women. From 2010 to 2019, the number of new ovarian cancer cases decreased slightly each year, as did the number of deaths from ovarian cancer from 2011 to 2020.

Symptoms of Ovarian Cancer

Early-stage ovarian cancer may not cause any symptoms. When symptoms do appear, the cancer is often advanced. Symptoms can include:

- bloating
- pelvic or abdominal pain
- trouble eating or feeling full quickly
- urinary symptoms (urgency or frequency)

Advanced symptoms may include:

- fatigue
- upset stomach
- back pain
- pain during sex
- constipation
- menstrual changes

These symptoms can be caused by conditions other than ovarian cancer, but it is important to see a doctor if you experience any of them.

Risk Factors for Ovarian, Fallopian Tube, and Primary Peritoneal Cancers

- **Family history**. A family history of ovarian, fallopian tube, or primary peritoneal cancers increases risk.
- **Inherited risk**. Certain gene mutations, such as *BRCA1* and *BRCA2*, increase the risk of these cancers. Syndromes like familial site-specific ovarian cancer syndrome and Lynch syndrome also increase risk.
- **Hormone replacement therapy (HRT)**. Slightly increases the risk of ovarian cancer, particularly in women who have recently used HRT.
- **Weight and height**. Being overweight or obese is linked to an increased risk of ovarian cancer, as is being tall.
- **Endometriosis**. Increases the risk of ovarian cancer.

Reducing Risk for Ovarian, Fallopian Tube, and Primary Peritoneal Cancers

- **Oral contraceptives**. Taking oral contraceptives reduces the risk of ovarian cancer. The longer they are used, the lower the risk.
- **Tubal ligation**. Surgery to close the fallopian tubes reduces the risk of ovarian cancer.
- **Giving birth**. Having children decreases the risk of ovarian cancer, with the risk further reduced for women who have more than one child.
- **Salpingectomy**. Removing one or both fallopian tubes lowers the risk of ovarian cancer.
- **Breastfeeding**. Reduces the risk of ovarian cancer, with longer breastfeeding durations associated with greater risk reduction.
- **Risk-reducing salpingo-oophorectomy**. Women with a high risk of ovarian cancer, such as those with *BRCA1* or *BRCA2* mutations, may choose to have surgery to remove the fallopian tubes and ovaries to reduce their risk.[4]

Section 15.7 | Kidney and Urinary Tract Cancers

BLADDER CANCER

What Is Bladder Cancer?

Bladder cancer occurs when bladder cells grow uncontrollably. The bladder is a hollow, balloon-shaped organ in the lower abdomen that stores urine. Its muscular wall allows it to expand to store urine and contract to expel urine from the body. The kidneys, located on each side of the backbone above the waist, filter and clean the

[4] "Ovarian, Fallopian Tube, and Primary Peritoneal Cancers Prevention (PDQ®)–Patient Version," National Cancer Institute (NCI), October 25, 2023. Available online. URL: www.cancer.gov/types/ovarian/patient/ovarian-prevention-pdq. Accessed April 25, 2024.

blood, producing urine that travels through the ureters to the bladder. The urine is then held in the bladder until it passes through the urethra and exits the body.

Signs and Symptoms of Bladder Cancer

Many bladder cancer symptoms are similar to those of less serious conditions. These are the warning signs you should not ignore:

- blood in the urine (hematuria)
- frequent urination
- painful urination
- back pain
- pelvic pain

If you experience any of these symptoms, consult your doctor to determine the cause.

Causes and Risk Factors of Bladder Cancer

Using tobacco, especially smoking cigarettes, is a major risk factor for bladder cancer. Other risk factors include:

- exposure to certain chemicals
- chronic bladder inflammation
- family history of bladder cancer
- previous cancer treatment with certain drugs or radiation[1]

What Can You Do to Reduce Your Risk of Bladder Cancer?

Bladder problems are more common among smokers, and smoking increases the risk of bladder cancer. If you smoke, take steps to quit.[2]

[1] "What Is Bladder Cancer?" National Cancer Institute (NCI), February 16, 2023. Available online. URL: www.cancer.gov/types/bladder. Accessed April 22, 2024.

[2] National Institute on Aging (NIA), "15 Tips to Keep Your Bladder Healthy," National Institutes of Health (NIH), January 24, 2022. Available online. URL: www.nia.nih.gov/health/bladder-health-and-incontinence/15-tips-keep-your-bladder-healthy. Accessed April 22, 2024.

KIDNEY AND RENAL PELVIS CANCERS

What Are Kidney and Renal Pelvis Cancers?

Cancer is a disease in which cells in the body grow out of control. When cancer starts in the kidney, it is called "kidney and renal pelvis cancer." The most common type of kidney cancer is renal cell carcinoma.

Signs and Symptoms of Kidney and Renal Pelvis Cancers

A person with kidney or renal pelvis cancer may have one or more of the following symptoms:

- blood in the urine
- a lump or swelling in the kidney area or abdomen
- lower back pain or pain in the side that does not go away
- frequent fatigue
- recurring fever
- loss of appetite
- unexplained weight loss
- blocked bowels
- a general feeling of poor health

Other conditions can also cause these symptoms. If you have any of these symptoms, talk to your doctor.

Causes and Risk Factors of Kidney and Renal Pelvis Cancers

Risk factors for kidney and renal pelvis cancers include:

- smoking
- being overweight or obese
- high blood pressure (HBP; possibly due to the condition or the medications used to treat it)
- long-term use of certain pain medications
- genetic conditions
- chronic hepatitis C infection
- kidney stones
- sickle cell trait (associated with renal medullary carcinoma)

- exposure to trichloroethylene (a chemical used to remove grease from metal)

What Can You Do to Reduce Your Risk?

To lower your risk of kidney and renal pelvis cancers, follow these lifestyle activities:

- Do not smoke, or quit if you do.
- Maintain a healthy weight.
- Eat a healthy diet.
- Be physically active.
- Be cautious with chemical exposure, especially trichloroethylene, which is used in some metalworking jobs.[3]

Section 15.8 | Blood and Bone Marrow Cancer

WHAT IS ADULT ACUTE MYELOID LEUKEMIA?

Adult acute myeloid leukemia (AML) is a cancer of the blood and bone marrow in which the bone marrow produces numerous abnormal blood cells. AML is the most common type of acute leukemia in adults and usually progresses rapidly if left untreated. It is also called "acute myelogenous leukemia" and "acute nonlymphocytic leukemia." AML affects red blood cells, white blood cells, and platelets.

Normally, the bone marrow produces blood stem cells (immature cells) that mature into blood cells over time. These blood stem cells mature into cells in the myeloid line or the lymphoid line. AML occurs due to a problem with blood stem cell development in the myeloid line. Myeloid stem cells go through several developmental stages in the bone marrow before maturing into:

- red blood cells that carry oxygen and other substances to all tissues of the body

[3] "Kidney Cancer Basics," Centers for Disease Control and Prevention (CDC), November 6, 2023. Available online. URL: www.cdc.gov/kidney-cancer/about. Accessed July 22, 2024.

- granulocytes and other types of white blood cells that help the body's immune system respond to infection, allergens, and inflammation
- platelets that help stop bleeding by forming clots

In AML, the number of immature white blood cells called "myeloblasts" or "myeloid blasts" increases. These myeloblasts are abnormal and do not develop into healthy white blood cells. As the number of these leukemia cells increases in the blood and bone marrow, there is less room for healthy platelets, red blood cells, and other white blood cells, leading to easy bleeding, anemia, and infection.

Leukemia cells can spread to other parts of the body, including the central nervous system (CNS), skin, and gums. Sometimes, leukemia cells form a solid tumor called a "myeloid sarcoma" or "chloroma."

SIGNS AND SYMPTOMS OF ADULT ACUTE MYELOID LEUKEMIA

The early signs and symptoms of AML may resemble those of the flu or other common diseases. Check with your doctor if you experience:

- weakness or feeling tired
- fever
- infection
- paleness or loss of normal skin color
- bleeding

Less common signs or symptoms may be caused by clusters of leukemia cells in the CNS or testicles or a tumor of myeloid cells called a "chloroma."

Symptoms of acute leukemia often develop between four and six weeks before diagnosis.

CAUSES AND RISK FACTORS OF ADULT ACUTE MYELOID LEUKEMIA

Smoking, previous chemotherapy treatment, and exposure to radiation may increase the risk of AML. AML is caused by changes in how blood stem cells function, particularly how they grow and divide into new cells. A risk factor is anything that increases the chance of developing a disease. Some risk factors for AML, such as smoking, can be modified, while others, like genetics and age, cannot.

Risk factors for AML include:

- smoking
- being male
- older age
- previous chemotherapy or radiation therapy
- exposure to environmental radiation (such as nuclear radiation) or the chemical benzene
- personal history of a blood disorder, such as myelodysplastic syndrome
- certain syndromes or inherited disorders

Having one or more of these risk factors does not mean you will develop AML. Many people with risk factors never develop AML, while others with no known risk factors do.[1]

WHAT CAN YOU DO TO REDUCE YOUR RISK?

Quitting smoking at any age can lead to substantial gains in life expectancy compared to continuing to smoke. Quitting smoking at the time of a cancer diagnosis also reduces the risk of death.[2]

[1] "Acute Myeloid Leukemia Treatment (PDQ®)–Patient Version," National Cancer Institute (NCI), March 6, 2024. Available online. URL: www.cancer.gov/types/leukemia/patient/adult-aml-treatment-pdq#_36. Accessed April 22, 2024.

[2] "Tobacco," National Cancer Institute (NCI), January 23, 2017. Available online. URL: www.cancer.gov/about-cancer/causes-prevention/risk/tobacco. Accessed April 22, 2024.

Chapter 16 | Smoking and Respiratory Diseases

Chapter Contents

Section 16.1 | The Effects of Cigarette Smoking on Lung Health

Cigarette smoking can cause immediate damage to your health. Each puff of cigarette smoke contains a mix of over 7,000 chemicals. When you breathe this in, the smoke hits your lungs quickly, and the blood carried to the rest of your body contains these toxic chemicals. Because tobacco smoke contains carbon monoxide, this deadly gas displaces the oxygen in your blood, depriving your organs of the oxygen they need.

Other chemicals found in cigarette smoke include acrolein, which can cause lung damage and, even in low amounts, can cause a sore throat in 10 minutes. Cigarettes may also contain bronchodilators—chemicals that open up the airways of the lungs and could increase the amount of dangerous chemicals absorbed by the lungs.

EFFECTS ON DIFFERENT AGE GROUPS

Cigarette smoking can have major consequences on the lungs at all ages. Babies whose mothers smoked during pregnancy may have lungs that develop abnormally, and teens who smoke cigarettes can develop smaller, weaker lungs that never grow to full size and never perform at their peak capacity. Additionally, smoking can destroy the cilia—tiny hairs in your airway that keep dirt and mucus out of your lungs. When these cilia are destroyed, you develop what is known as a "smoker's cough," a chronic cough often seen in long-term or daily smokers.

CHRONIC OBSTRUCTIVE PULMONARY DISEASE

Lung damage due to smoking does not end there. Eight out of ten cases of chronic obstructive pulmonary disease (COPD) are caused by smoking. People with COPD experience difficulty breathing and eventually die because of a lack of air. There is no cure for COPD. Furthermore, nearly all lung cancer—the top cause of cancer death in both men and women—is caused by smoking. Smokers are 20 times more likely to develop lung cancer than nonsmokers.

In addition to lung cancer, smoking can lead to other respiratory cancers, such as those affecting the:

- oropharynx (the back of the mouth, including parts of the tongue, the soft palate, the side and back of the throat, and the tonsils)
- larynx (the voice box)
- trachea (the windpipe)
- bronchus (one of two large airways that connect the trachea to the lungs)

NOT JUST CIGARETTES: OTHER TOBACCO PRODUCTS AND LUNG HEALTH

While cigarettes, given their high rate of use, addictive nature, and toxic mix of chemicals, are the most dangerous tobacco product, any tobacco product you inhale could cause lung damage. Cigar smoking can increase the risk of COPD and lead to cancers of the lung, oral cavity, and larynx, among other cancers.

Electronic nicotine delivery systems (ENDS), such as electronic cigarettes (e-cigarettes), are still relatively new tobacco products and are still being evaluated for their effects on health. But e-cigarette use—or vaping—may be harmful to your lungs. Some e-cigarette aerosols have been found to contain some of the same chemicals in cigarettes, including the lung irritant acrolein and formaldehyde, which may adversely affect the throat. Flavoring chemicals are considered safe for eating but could be harmful when inhaled. Buttery flavors such as caramel, toffee, and chocolate contain the chemicals diacetyl and acetoin, which can be harmful to your lungs. Additionally, fruit-flavored e-cigarettes can have higher concentrations of a chemical called "acrylonitrile," which is a known respiratory irritant.

HOW YOU CAN PROTECT YOUR LUNGS FROM TOBACCO

Your lungs are one of your body's filtration systems, taking in air from the atmosphere, adding oxygen to the blood for circulation throughout the body, and expelling excess carbon dioxide. When tobacco is inhaled, it interferes with this delicate balance. The best way to ensure lung health is to never start using tobacco. If you are an addicted smoker, the sooner you quit, the sooner your lungs can begin to heal. Quitting smoking can lower the risk of getting cancer. In fact, when you quit smoking, your risk of:

- cancer of the larynx is reduced immediately
- lung cancer drops by 50 percent 10 years after quitting
- mouth and throat cancers drop by 50 percent five years after quitting

Anyone who quits smoking will experience better overall health. Just 12 hours after quitting, the carbon monoxide level in your blood drops to normal, allowing more oxygen to circulate to your organs.[1]

Section 16.2 | Asthma

WHAT IS ASTHMA?

Asthma is a chronic disease that affects the airways of the lungs. During an asthma attack, the airways (tubes that carry air to your lungs) become swollen, making it hard to breathe. As the walls of the airways swell, they narrow, and less air gets in and out of the lungs. Cells in the airways can produce more mucus (a sticky, thick liquid) than usual, which can make breathing even harder.

SYMPTOMS OF AN ASTHMA ATTACK

- coughing
- shortness of breath or trouble breathing
- wheezing
- tightness or pain in the chest

[1] "Keep Your Air Clear: How Tobacco Can Harm Your Lungs," U.S. Food and Drug Administration (FDA), May 4, 2020. Available online. URL: www.fda.gov/tobacco-products/health-effects-tobacco-use/keep-your-air-clear-how-tobacco-can-harm-your-lungs. Accessed April 22, 2024.

Asthma attacks can be mild, moderate, serious, or even life-threatening.

SMOKING AND ASTHMA

If you have asthma, an asthma attack can occur when something irritates your airways and triggers an attack. Your triggers might be different from other people's triggers.

Tobacco smoke is a common trigger for asthma. Tobacco smoke—including secondhand smoke—is unhealthy for everyone, especially people with asthma. Secondhand smoke is a mixture of gases and fine particles that include:

- smoke from burning tobacco products, such as cigarettes, cigars, or pipes
- smoke that has been exhaled (breathed out) by someone who smokes

Secondhand smoke contains more than 7,000 chemicals, including hundreds that are toxic and about 70 that can cause cancer. If you have asthma, it is important to avoid exposure to secondhand smoke. If you are among the 21 percent of U.S. adults who have asthma and smoke, get help to quit smoking. Talk to your doctor about treatments that can help you, or call 1-800-QUIT-NOW.

PREVENTING ASTHMA ATTACKS

If you or a family member has asthma, you can manage it with the help of your health-care provider (e.g., by taking your medicines exactly as your doctor tells you) and by avoiding your triggers. To prevent asthma attacks, stay far away from tobacco smoke. Some other helpful tips are:

- **Do not smoke or allow others to smoke in your home or car.** Opening a window does not protect you from smoke.
- **If your state still allows smoking in public areas, look for restaurants and other places that do not allow smoking.** No-smoking sections in the same restaurant with smoking sections do not protect adequately

from secondhand smoke—even if there is a filter or ventilation system.
- **Make sure your children's day care centers and schools are tobacco-free**. For schools, a tobacco-free campus policy means no tobacco use or advertising on school property is allowed by anyone at any time. This includes off-campus school events.
- **Teach children to stay away from secondhand smoke**. Be a good role model by not smoking.

TREATING ASTHMA

There is no cure for asthma. However, to help control your asthma and avoid attacks:
- Take your medicine exactly as your doctor tells you.
- Stay away from things that can trigger an attack.

Not everyone with asthma takes the same medicine. Some medicines can be inhaled, and some can be taken as a pill. There are two kinds of asthma medicines:
- quick-relief (can help control symptoms of an asthma attack)
- long-term control (can help you have fewer and milder attacks, but they do not help you while you are having an asthma attack)[1]

Section 16.3 | **Chronic Obstructive Pulmonary Disease**

WHAT IS CHRONIC OBSTRUCTIVE PULMONARY DISEASE?

Chronic obstructive pulmonary disease (COPD) refers to a group of diseases that cause airflow blockage and breathing-related problems. COPD includes emphysema, chronic bronchitis, and, in some cases, asthma.

---

[1] "Asthma and Secondhand Smoke," Centers for Disease Control and Prevention (CDC), October 13, 2023. Available online. URL: www.cdc.gov/tobacco/campaign/tips/diseases/secondhand-smoke-asthma.html. Accessed April 22, 2024.

With COPD, less air flows through the airways that carry air in and out of your lungs. This happens because of one or more of the following:

- The airways and tiny air sacs in the lungs lose their ability to stretch and shrink back.
- The walls between many of the air sacs are destroyed.
- The walls of the airways become thick and inflamed (irritated and swollen).
- The airways make more mucus than usual. The mucus can clog airways and block airflow.

In the early stages of COPD, there may be no symptoms or only mild symptoms. As COPD worsens, the symptoms may become more severe. The severity of COPD symptoms depends on the amount of damage to the lungs. Continued smoking leads to lung damage worsening faster than not smoking.

SMOKING, SECONDHAND SMOKE EXPOSURE, AND CHRONIC OBSTRUCTIVE PULMONARY DISEASE

Cigarette smoking is a common cause of COPD. Smoking causes as many as 8 out of 10 COPD-related deaths. However, as many as one out of four Americans with COPD never smoked cigarettes.

Smoking and secondhand smoke exposure during childhood and teenage years can slow lung growth and development, increasing the risk of developing COPD in adulthood.

The best way to prevent COPD is to never start smoking. If you smoke, quitting is the most important action you can take. It is also important to avoid secondhand smoke. Secondhand smoke is smoke from burning tobacco products, such as cigarettes, cigars, or pipes.

QUITTING SMOKING CAN PROTECT PEOPLE FROM CHRONIC OBSTRUCTIVE PULMONARY DISEASE

Quitting smoking is one of the most important actions people can take to improve their health. This is true for all people who smoke, regardless of their age, how long they have smoked, or how much they smoke. Quitting smoking also reduces the risk of developing COPD. For patients diagnosed with COPD, quitting smoking slows the disease's progression and reduces the loss of lung function over time.[1]

[1] "Chronic Obstructive Pulmonary Disease (COPD)," Centers for Disease Control and Prevention (CDC), May 15, 2024. Available online. URL: www.cdc.gov/tobacco/about/cigarettes-and-copd.html. Accessed July 22, 2024.

Chapter 17 | Smoking and Cardiovascular Diseases

Chapter Contents

Smoking cigarettes can harm nearly any part of your body, including your heart and blood vessels (cardiovascular system). When breathed in, the toxic mix of more than 7,000 chemicals in cigarette smoke can interfere with important processes that keep your body functioning normally. One of these processes is delivering oxygen-rich blood to your heart and the rest of your body.

When you breathe, your lungs take in oxygen and deliver it to your heart, which pumps this oxygen-rich blood to the rest of your body through the blood vessels. However, when you breathe in cigarette smoke, the blood that is distributed to the rest of the body becomes contaminated with the smoke's chemicals. These chemicals can damage your heart and blood vessels, leading to cardiovascular disease (CVD)—the leading cause of all deaths in the United States.

CARDIOVASCULAR CONDITIONS RESULTING FROM SMOKING

Smoking cigarettes can permanently damage your heart and blood vessels, leading to CVD. CVD refers to multiple conditions affecting the heart and/or blood vessels. Some of these conditions include the following:

- coronary heart disease, or the narrowing of blood vessels carrying blood to the heart
- hypertension (high blood pressure (HBP))
- heart attack
- stroke
- aneurysms (a bulge or weakness in an artery)
- peripheral artery disease (PAD)

Smoking cigarettes can also cause CVD by changing your blood chemistry. These changes can cause plaque—a waxy substance comprised of cholesterol, scar tissue, calcium, fat, and other material—to build up in your arteries, the major blood vessels that carry blood from your heart to your body. This plaque buildup can lead to a disease called "atherosclerosis."

When the chemicals in cigarette smoke cause atherosclerosis and thickened blood in the arteries, it becomes more difficult for blood cells to move through arteries and other blood vessels to reach vital organs such as the heart and brain. This can create blood clots and ultimately lead to a heart attack or stroke, even death.

Other rare but serious cardiovascular conditions caused by smoking include:

- **Peripheral artery disease (PAD; and peripheral vascular disease).** A condition in which the narrowing of blood vessels results in insufficient blood flow to arms, legs, hands, and feet. Smoking is the leading preventable cause of this condition, which can result in amputation.
- **Abdominal aortic aneurysm.** A bulge that forms in an area of the aorta—the main artery that distributes blood through the body—that sits in the abdomen. When an abdominal aortic aneurysm bursts, it can result in sudden death. More women than men die from aortic aneurysms, and nearly all deaths from this condition are caused by smoking.

MORTALITY FROM CARDIOVASCULAR DISEASE CAUSED BY SMOKING

According to the American Heart Association (AHA), CVD accounts for about 800,000 U.S. deaths every year, making it the leading cause of all deaths in the United States. Of those, nearly 20 percent are due to cigarette smoking.

SECONDHAND SMOKE AND CORONARY HEART DISEASE

While smoking is a direct cause of CVD and death, you could be at risk even if you do not smoke cigarettes. People who do not smoke cigarettes but who are regularly exposed to secondhand smoke have a 25–30 percent increased risk of coronary heart disease compared to those not exposed. In fact, 30,000 U.S. coronary heart disease deaths per year are caused by secondhand smoke. Secondhand smoke exposure also increases your risk of having a heart attack or stroke.

BENEFITS OF QUITTING SMOKING FOR HEART HEALTH

The best way to safeguard your heart from smoking-related disease and death is to never start using cigarettes. However, if you do smoke, the earlier you quit, the better. Quitting smoking benefits your heart and cardiovascular system now and in the future:

- 20 minutes after you quit smoking, your heart rate drops
- just 12 hours after quitting smoking, the carbon monoxide level in your blood drops to normal, allowing more oxygen to vital organs such as your heart
- within four years of quitting, your risk of stroke drops to that of lifetime nonsmokers

STRATEGIES FOR QUITTING SMOKING TO PROTECT YOUR HEART

Although quitting smoking is difficult, it is achievable. The U.S. Food and Drug Administration (FDA)-approved nicotine replacement therapy (NRT) may help you on your quit journey. NRTs are proven safe and effective in helping you quit smoking by delivering measured amounts of nicotine without the toxic chemicals found in cigarette smoke. Many people who smoke find that FDA-approved NRTs help them get through the first steps of quitting by reducing cravings and symptoms of withdrawal.

If you smoke and are concerned about your heart and cardiovascular health, consult with your health-care provider about NRTs or other ways to quit to help protect your heart.[1]

Section 17.2 | **Abdominal Aortic Aneurysms**

WHAT IS ABDOMINAL AORTIC ANEURYSM?

The aorta is your body's main artery. An artery is a blood vessel (or tube) that carries blood from your heart. The aorta carries blood from your heart to your abdomen, pelvis, and legs.

[1] "How Smoking Affects Heart Health," U.S. Food and Drug Administration (FDA), November 9, 2021. Available online. URL: www.fda.gov/tobacco-products/health-effects-tobacco-use/how-smoking-affects-heart-health. Accessed April 23, 2024.

If the wall of your aorta is weak, it can start to bulge. This balloon-like bulge is called an "aneurysm." An abdominal aortic aneurysm (AAA) is an aneurysm that happens in the part of the aorta running through the abdomen.

SIGNS AND SYMPTOMS OF ABDOMINAL AORTIC ANEURYSM

Abdominal aortic aneurysms do not usually cause symptoms until they are a medical emergency. Blood vessels such as the aorta can bulge out slowly over time, so it is important to talk with your doctor about AAA to see if you need to get tested. Although people with an AAA may not have any symptoms, some people may notice:

- back pain
- a pulse you can feel near or below your belly button
- dull ache or pain in the belly or side of your belly
- discolored skin or sores on feet and toes (this is rare)

When an AAA ruptures or starts to leak blood, it is a medical emergency since blood loss from the aorta can lead to death. Some symptoms of a ruptured AAA include:

- sudden pain in your lower back, abdomen, or legs—usually the pain is severe
- fast heart rate
- low blood pressure
- nausea and vomiting
- clammy (sweaty) skin

If you think you have a ruptured aneurysm, call 911 or have someone take you to the closest emergency room. You will need to have life-saving surgery right away.

CAUSES AND RISK FACTORS OF ABDOMINAL AORTIC ANEURYSM

Men over age 65 who have smoked at any point in their lives have the highest risk of AAA. Both men and women can have AAA, but it is more common in men. Risk factors for AAA include the following:

- smoking, both if you smoke now or you smoked in the past

- family history—for example, if a parent or sibling had AAA
- older age, especially 65 years or older
- being white
- having other aneurysms, such as thoracic aortic aneurysm (similar to AAA but in the chest instead of the abdomen)
- high blood pressure (HBP) or high cholesterol
- heart disease or vascular disease (problems with blood vessels)

PREVENTION OF ABDOMINAL AORTIC ANEURYSM

Quitting smoking is the most important thing you can do to lower your risk for AAA. If you smoke, now is the time to quit! Call 1-800-QUIT-NOW (1-800-784-8669) for free support and help making a plan to quit.[1]

Section 17.3 | Atherosclerosis

WHAT IS ATHEROSCLEROSIS?

Atherosclerosis is a common condition that develops when a sticky substance called "plaque" builds up inside your arteries. Disease linked to atherosclerosis is the leading cause of death in the United States.

CAUSES AND RISK FACTORS

Risk factors are conditions or habits that make a person more likely to develop a disease. Nearly half of Americans have high blood pressure (HBP) or unhealthy cholesterol levels, or they smoke. These are key risk factors that can trigger the start of plaque buildup.

[1] Office of Disease Prevention and Health Promotion (ODPHP), "Talk to Your Doctor about Abdominal Aortic Aneurysm," U.S. Department of Health and Human Services (HHS), March 30, 2023. Available online. URL: https://health.gov/myhealthfinder/health-conditions/heart-health/talk-your-doctor-about-abdominal-aortic-aneurysm#the-basics-tab. Accessed April 23, 2024.

What Causes Atherosclerosis?

Atherosclerosis develops slowly as cholesterol, fat, blood cells, and other substances in your blood form plaque. When the plaque builds up, it causes your arteries to narrow, reducing the supply of oxygen-rich blood to tissues of vital organs in the body.

Atherosclerosis can affect most of the arteries in the body, including arteries in the heart, brain, arms, legs, pelvis, and kidneys. It has different names based on which arteries are affected:

- **Coronary artery disease (CAD).** Plaque buildup in the arteries of your heart.
- **Peripheral artery disease (PAD).** Plaque buildup in the arteries of the legs, arms, or pelvis.
- **Carotid artery disease.** Plaque buildup in the neck arteries, reducing blood flow to the brain.
- **Renal artery stenosis.** Plaque buildup in the arteries that supply blood to your kidneys.
- **Vertebral artery disease.** Atherosclerosis in the arteries that supply blood to the back of the brain.
- **Mesenteric artery ischemia.** Plaque buildup in the arteries that supply the intestines with blood.

What Raises the Risk of Atherosclerosis?

The risk factors for plaque buildup are often linked. For example, smoking and a lack of regular physical activity raise the risk of unhealthy cholesterol levels, which can lead to plaque buildup.

Other common risk factors for plaque buildup include:

- **High blood pressure.** Over time, HBP can damage artery walls, allowing plaque to build up.
- **Diabetes.** High blood sugar can damage the inner layers of the arteries, causing plaque buildup.
- **Metabolic syndrome.** High levels of cholesterol and triglycerides in your blood increase your risk.
- **Unhealthy diet.** Eating many foods high in saturated fats can increase your cholesterol levels.
- **Family history.** Your genes may increase your risk, especially if you have a common inherited cholesterol disorder called "familial hypercholesterolemia."

- **Inflammatory diseases.** Conditions such as rheumatoid arthritis (RA) and psoriasis can lead to high levels of inflammation, irritating your blood vessels and leading to plaque buildup.
- **Older age.** For most people, plaque buildup starts in childhood and gets worse as they get older. In men, the risk increases after 45. In women, the risk increases after 55. The risk for women is even higher if you have endometriosis or polycystic ovary syndrome or if you have gestational diabetes or preeclampsia during pregnancy.

SYMPTOMS AND COMPLICATIONS

Reduced blood flow can lead to symptoms such as angina. If a plaque bursts, a blood clot may form that may block the artery completely or travel to other parts of the body. Blockages, either complete or incomplete, can cause complications, including heart attack, stroke, vascular dementia, erectile dysfunction, or limb loss. Atherosclerosis can cause death and disability.

Atherosclerosis leads to a poor oxygen-rich blood supply and symptoms that can affect quality of life (QOL). Symptoms depend on which arteries are affected and how much blood flow is blocked.

- **Coronary artery disease.** Chest pain (angina), cold sweats, dizziness, extreme tiredness, heart palpitations (feeling that your heart is racing), shortness of breath, nausea, and weakness.
- **Peripheral artery disease.** Pain, aching, heaviness, or cramping in the legs when walking or climbing stairs, with symptoms typically going away after rest.
- **Vertebral artery disease.** Problems with thinking and memory, weakness or numbness on one side of the body or face, vision trouble, and transient ischemic attack (TIA), commonly called a "mini-stroke."
- **Mesenteric artery ischemia.** Severe pain following meals, weight loss, and diarrhea.
- **Erectile dysfunction (ED).** An early warning sign that a man may be at higher risk for atherosclerosis and its complications.

You may not notice other symptoms until plaque buildup causes serious problems. Seeing your doctor regularly is important, as they may be able to find plaque buildup before it gets serious. For example:

- **Carotid artery disease.** Plaque buildup in the arteries of the neck can cause a bruit, a whooshing sound that your doctor hears when using a stethoscope. Severe symptoms of a bruit include a transient ischemic attack (TIA).
- **Renal artery stenosis.** Using a stethoscope, doctors may hear a bruit in your belly, an early sign of plaque buildup in the arteries that deliver blood to the kidneys. As the disease worsens, it can cause HBP, extreme tiredness, loss of appetite, nausea, swelling in the hands or feet, and itchiness or numbness.

Talk to your doctor about your symptoms and whether you have risk factors for atherosclerosis.

PREVENTION AND MANAGEMENT

Taking action to control your risk factors can help prevent or slow down plaque buildup. If lifestyle changes are not enough, your doctor may prescribe medicine to control your atherosclerosis risk factors. Take all of your medicines as your doctor advises.

Heart-Healthy Lifestyle

A heart-healthy lifestyle starts early in life. Atherosclerosis often begins in childhood and continues to develop throughout life. Heart-healthy living—never smoking, eating healthy, and being physically active—starting in childhood and continuing throughout life can prevent atherosclerosis and its complications. Help your kids follow a heart-healthy lifestyle and encourage them not to smoke or vape.

Medicines to Control Blood Cholesterol Levels

Doctors now have a range of medicines they can prescribe to manage blood cholesterol levels. Your doctor may prescribe a statin or another medicine, depending on several factors: your risk for complications, such as heart attack and stroke; whether you have diabetes; your age; and your cholesterol levels. High levels of "bad" cholesterol are an important risk factor for plaque buildup.

Talk with your health-care team about whether medicines can help you reduce your risk for plaque buildup. Even if you take medicine as part of your treatment plan, be sure to continue your healthy lifestyle changes.

Treating Other Health Conditions

Certain medical conditions are risk factors for plaque buildup and complications of atherosclerosis. Your health-care team can help treat conditions such as chronic kidney disease, diabetes, HBP, high blood triglycerides, and infections, such as HIV, hepatitis C, and bacterial infections.

Make an appointment with your health-care team to discuss how to keep your heart healthy. Talk to your doctor about your blood pressure, cholesterol, and blood glucose (sugar) numbers.[1]

Section 17.4 | Coronary Heart Disease and Heart Attacks

WHAT IS CORONARY HEART DISEASE?

Heart disease encompasses various conditions that affect the heart's structure and function. It is the leading cause of death in the United States. Coronary heart disease, also known as "coronary artery disease" or "ischemic heart disease," occurs when the arteries of the heart cannot deliver enough oxygen-rich blood to the heart. According to the Centers for Disease Control and Prevention (CDC), approximately 20.5 million U.S. adults have coronary artery disease (CAD), making it the most common type of heart disease in the country.

[1] "Atherosclerosis," National Heart, Lung, and Blood Institute (NHLBI), March 24, 2022. Available online. URL: www.nhlbi.nih.gov/health/atherosclerosis. Accessed July 22, 2024.

Coronary artery disease affects the larger coronary arteries on the heart's surface, while coronary microvascular disease affects the tiny arteries within the heart muscle. The latter is more common in women.

The cause of coronary heart disease varies. Coronary artery disease is often caused by cholesterol buildup inside the coronary arteries, forming plaque that can block blood flow. Coronary microvascular disease occurs when damage occurs to the inner walls of the heart's small blood vessels. Most coronary heart disease is preventable with a heart-healthy lifestyle and medications.

Symptoms of coronary heart disease differ among individuals. Many people have no symptoms until they experience chest pain, a heart attack, or cardiac arrest. If you have coronary heart disease, you may need lifestyle changes, medications, surgery, or a combination of these to manage your condition and prevent serious problems.

SYMPTOMS OF CORONARY HEART DISEASE

Sometimes coronary heart disease is silent, making it hard to diagnose until complications arise. This highlights the importance of prevention.

CAUSES AND RISK FACTORS OF CORONARY HEART DISEASE

What Causes Coronary Heart Disease?

Coronary heart disease can stem from plaque buildup or problems with the heart's blood vessels. Preventive measures from early life can mitigate risk factors.

PLAQUE BUILDUP

Atherosclerosis, the buildup of plaque in the arteries, can block blood flow to the heart muscle. This is the primary cause of obstructive CAD. Small plaques can also build up in the heart's small blood vessels, causing coronary microvascular disease.

PROBLEMS WITH BLOOD VESSEL FUNCTION

Blood vessels may not widen to allow more blood flow to the heart during physical activity or stress, potentially narrowing instead.

Chronic inflammation, high blood pressure (HBP), or diabetes may cause such problems, leading to coronary heart disease. Damage to the inner walls of coronary arteries can also cause vasospasm, temporarily blocking blood flow to the heart.

Risk Factors for Coronary Heart Disease

The risk of coronary heart disease increases with the number and severity of risk factors. Some factors, such as HBP and cholesterol, can be managed through lifestyle changes, while others, like age and family history, cannot be changed.

LIFESTYLE HABITS

Unhealthy habits, such as smoking, physical inactivity, poor sleep, stress, and unhealthy eating patterns, can lead to plaque buildup in the heart's blood vessels.

AGE

Plaque buildup increases with age. Men's risk rises substantially around age 45, and women's risk increases after menopause, around age 55.

ENVIRONMENT AND OCCUPATION

Air pollution can increase the risk of coronary heart disease, especially in older adults, women, and people with diabetes or obesity. Work-related stress, exposure to toxins, prolonged sitting, and irregular or night shifts also raise risk.

FAMILY HISTORY AND GENETICS

A family history of early heart disease is a significant risk factor, especially if a close relative was diagnosed before age 55 (men) or 65 (women). Certain genes are linked to higher coronary heart disease risk.

OTHER MEDICAL CONDITIONS

Conditions such as atherosclerosis, congenital coronary artery defects, high blood LDL cholesterol, HBP, and high blood triglycerides increase coronary heart disease risk. Autoimmune diseases, chronic kidney disease, diabetes, HIV/AIDS, mental health conditions, metabolic syndrome, obesity, and sleep disorders also contribute to risk.

RACE OR ETHNICITY

Heart disease is the leading cause of death for most racial and ethnic groups in the United States. South Asians have a higher risk of coronary heart disease and complications.

SEX

Obstructive coronary artery disease is more common in men, while nonobstructive coronary artery disease is more common in women and harder to diagnose. Women with chest discomfort or shortness of breath during physical activity should seek tests for nonobstructive coronary artery disease or coronary microvascular disease.

PREVENTION OF CORONARY HEART DISEASE

Your provider may recommend adopting lifelong heart-healthy lifestyle changes, such as:

- quitting smoking to prevent blood vessel damage and tightening
- choosing heart-healthy foods, including fruits, vegetables, and whole grains, while limiting saturated fats, sodium, added sugars, and alcohol
- being physically active to manage coronary heart disease risk factors such as high cholesterol, HBP, or obesity
- getting enough good-quality sleep, aiming for 7–9 hours per night
- maintaining a healthy weight to manage risk factors such as high cholesterol, diabetes, and HBP
- getting regular blood pressure and cholesterol checks
- controlling blood sugar levels to prevent blood vessel damage

- managing stress through relaxation and coping strategies[1]

WHAT IS A HEART ATTACK?

A heart attack, or myocardial infarction, occurs when the blood flow bringing oxygen to a part of the heart muscle is blocked. Without oxygen, the heart muscle begins to die. According to the CDC, more than 800,000 people in the United States have a heart attack each year. Heart attacks differ from cardiac arrest, where the heart suddenly stops beating. A heart attack can lead to sudden cardiac arrest.

SIGNS AND SYMPTOMS OF HEART ATTACKS

Heart attack symptoms vary and may not always involve severe chest pain. Symptoms can start slowly, be mild or severe, and come and go. They differ between men and women and from one heart attack to another. Common symptoms include:

- chest pain, heaviness, or discomfort
- pain or discomfort in arms, back, shoulders, neck, jaw, or above the belly button
- shortness of breath
- sweating without a clear reason
- unusual fatigue
- nausea and vomiting
- light-headedness or dizziness
- rapid or irregular heartbeat

Some people may have mild or no symptoms but still experience a heart attack.

When to Call 911

If you suspect a heart attack, call 911 immediately. Early intervention can limit heart damage and save lives. The 911 operator

[1] "Coronary Heart Disease," National Heart, Lung, and Blood Institute (NHLBI), December 20, 2023. Available online. URL: www.nhlbi.nih.gov/health/coronary-heart-disease. Accessed July 22, 2024.

or EMS personnel can provide lifesaving advice. An ambulance is the safest way to reach the hospital, ensuring prompt treatment.

CAUSES AND RISK FACTORS OF HEART ATTACKS

What Causes a Heart Attack?

Most heart attacks result from coronary artery disease, where plaque buildup narrows arteries and blocks blood flow. Plaques can rupture, forming blood clots that block blood flow to the heart. This blockage causes heart muscle death.

OTHER CAUSES OF A HEART ATTACK

Not all heart attacks result from atherosclerosis. Myocardial infarction in the absence of obstructive coronary artery disease (MINOCA) occurs when other heart and blood vessel conditions cause a heart attack. MINOCA is more common in women, younger people, and racial and ethnic minorities. Conditions causing MINOCA include:

- small plaques that can form blood clots
- sudden, serious spasms of coronary arteries
- coronary artery embolism, where a blood clot travels and blocks the artery
- spontaneous coronary artery dissection (SCAD), where a tear forms inside the artery

What Raises the Risk of a Heart Attack?

Risk factors for heart attacks include:

CONTROLLABLE FACTORS

- smoking
- unhealthy diet
- lack of physical activity
- high blood cholesterol
- high blood pressure
- high blood sugar or diabetes
- high blood triglycerides
- overweight and obesity

UNCONTROLLABLE FACTORS

- age (men over 45, women over 55)
- family history of early heart disease
- infections from bacteria and viruses

PREVENTION OF HEART ATTACK

Preventive measures include:

- heart-healthy eating
- maintaining a healthy weight
- managing stress
- regular physical activity
- quitting smoking[2]

Section 17.5 | **Peripheral Artery Disease**

WHAT IS PERIPHERAL ARTERY DISEASE?

In the United States, more than 8 million people aged 40 and older have peripheral artery disease (PAD). Also called "peripheral arterial disease," PAD is caused by atherosclerosis, or plaque buildup, which reduces blood flow in peripheral arteries. These arteries carry blood away from the heart to other body parts. This discussion focuses on the most common type of PAD, lower extremity PAD, which reduces blood flow to the legs and feet.

You may have lower extremity PAD if you experience muscle pain or weakness that begins with physical activity, such as walking, and stops within minutes after resting. About one in four people with PAD have these symptoms. However, some may experience different symptoms or none at all. If you smoke or have high blood pressure (HBP) or other risk factors for PAD, consult your healthcare provider about getting tested. It is important to be aware that if you have lower extremity PAD, you may also have plaque buildup

[2] "Heart Attack," National Heart, Lung, and Blood Institute (NHLBI), March 24, 2022. Available online. URL: www.nhlbi.nih.gov/health/heart-attack. Accessed July 22, 2024.

in other arteries leading to and from your heart and brain, putting you at higher risk of stroke or heart attack.

Early diagnosis and management of PAD can help treat your symptoms and reduce your risk for serious complications.

SIGNS AND SYMPTOMS OF PERIPHERAL ARTERY DISEASE

About one in four people with PAD experience common symptoms of the condition. More than half have nontypical symptoms, and about one in five do not report any symptoms. Regardless of symptoms, everyone with PAD shares a high risk of cardiovascular disease. Without treatment, PAD may cause sores, infections, and even the loss of a limb.

Common Symptoms of Peripheral Artery Disease

- pain, aching, heaviness, or cramping in your legs that begins with walking or climbing stairs and stops after resting (intermittent claudication); this pain is often in the calf but may also be in the buttocks, thigh, or foot
- toenails and leg hair may stop growing
- one foot may feel colder than the other
- the foot or leg may become pale, discolored, or blue
- leg weakness or numbness, affecting balance or walking
- pain or a pins-and-needles feeling in the leg or foot
- in severe PAD, pain in the leg and foot when at rest (critical limb ischemia)
- sores or wounds on the toes, feet, or legs that may appear, heal slowly, or not heal at all, potentially becoming infected

CAUSES AND RISK FACTORS OF PERIPHERAL ARTERY DISEASE

What Causes Peripheral Artery Disease?

Atherosclerosis is the main cause of PAD. It involves the buildup of plaque, a substance made of fat, cholesterol, fibrous tissue, and calcium, on the inner lining of arteries. Plaque can reduce or block the flow of oxygen-rich blood through arteries to vital organs and limbs.

What Raises the Risk of Peripheral Artery Disease?

Risk factors for lower extremity PAD include age, family history and genetics, lifestyle habits, other medical conditions, race, ethnicity, and sex. These risk factors are similar to those for coronary heart disease and carotid artery disease.

AGE

Peripheral artery disease can develop at any age, but the risk increases with age. Most people in the United States with PAD are aged 65 or older. In lower-income countries, the age group for PAD is younger (ages 45–49).

FAMILY HISTORY AND GENETICS

A family history of PAD, heart disease, stroke, or blood vessel disease raises your risk. Researchers are studying gene variations that increase the risk of PAD or worsen the disease. Certain gene variations are found in different types of atherosclerotic diseases, such as PAD, carotid artery disease, and coronary heart disease.

LIFESTYLE HABITS

Unhealthy lifestyle habits can lead to plaque buildup in the leg and foot arteries, causing PAD. These habits include smoking, physical inactivity, stress, and unhealthy eating patterns high in saturated fats.

OTHER MEDICAL CONDITIONS

Conditions that raise the risk of developing PAD include:

- diabetes
- chronic kidney disease
- blood clot disorders, such as thrombocytosis or antiphospholipid syndrome
- fibromuscular dysplasia
- high blood pressure
- metabolic syndrome
- obesity
- unhealthy blood cholesterol levels or high blood triglycerides

- history of preeclampsia or gestational diabetes during pregnancy

RACE OR ETHNICITY

African Americans have a higher risk of PAD and its complications, such as problems walking or limb loss. American Indian women have a higher risk of PAD than white or Asian-American women. Hispanic or Latino people and white people have similar risk levels, but lower extremity PAD rates are higher among sedentary Hispanic and Latino adults.

SEX

Men and women have similar risks of developing PAD, but it affects them differently. Women are more likely to have PAD without symptoms but also have more complications, such as walking problems.

PREVENTION OF PERIPHERAL ARTERY DISEASE

Your provider may recommend adopting lifelong heart-healthy lifestyle changes:

- **Quit smoking**. Smoking is the main risk factor for PAD. Quitting can reduce symptoms and risk of complications. Avoid secondhand smoke. Resources like Smoking and Your Heart and the NHLBI's Your Guide to a Healthy Heart provide basic information on quitting smoking. For free help, call the National Cancer Institute's Smoking Quitline at 1-877-44U-QUIT (1-877-448-7848).
- **Choose heart-healthy foods**. Follow the DASH (Dietary Approaches to Stop Hypertension) eating plan, which includes fruits, vegetables, and whole grains while limiting saturated fats, sodium, added sugars, and alcohol.
- **Aim for a healthy weight**. Losing even 3–5 percent of your current weight can help manage PAD risk factors such as high cholesterol and diabetes.

- **Get regular physical activity**. Staying active can help manage risk factors such as high cholesterol, HBP, and obesity. Consult your provider before starting an exercise program.
- **Manage stress.** Learn to manage stress, relax, get good-quality sleep, and cope with problems to improve emotional and physical health.

These measures can help prevent PAD and manage its risk factors effectively.[1]

Section 17.6 | Stroke

UNDERSTANDING STROKES

A stroke occurs when blood flow to the brain is blocked, or there is sudden bleeding in the brain.

Types of Strokes

There are two types of strokes:

1. **Ischemic stroke.** This occurs when blood flow to the brain is blocked. The brain cannot get oxygen and nutrients from the blood, and brain cells begin to die within minutes.
2. **Hemorrhagic stroke**. This occurs due to sudden bleeding in the brain. The leaked blood results in pressure on brain cells, damaging them.

Approximately 90 percent of strokes involve blocked blood vessels (ischemic), while the rest involve internal bleeding (hemorrhagic). Strokes are further classified based on where in the brain the blockage or bleeding occurs.

---

[1] "Peripheral Artery Disease," National Heart, Lung, and Blood Institute (NHLBI), March 24, 2022. Available online. URL: www.nhlbi.nih.gov/health/peripheral-artery-disease. Accessed July 22, 2024.

A stroke is a medical emergency that can cause lasting brain damage, long-term disability, or even death. Signs of a stroke range from mild weakness to paralysis or numbness on one side of the face or body. Other signs may include a sudden and severe headache, sudden weakness, trouble seeing, and trouble speaking or understanding speech.

The FAST Test

The FAST test can help you remember what to do if you think someone is having a stroke.

1. **F—Face**. Ask the person to smile. Does one side of the face droop?
2. **A—Arms**. Ask the person to raise both arms. Does one arm drift downward?
3. **S—Speech**. Ask the person to repeat a simple phrase. Is their speech slurred or strange?
4. **T—Time**. If you observe any of these signs, call 911 immediately. Early treatment is essential.

Immediate Action during a Stroke

If you think you or someone else may be having a stroke, call 911 immediately. Do not drive to the hospital or let someone else drive you. Call an ambulance so that medical personnel can begin life-saving treatment on the way to the emergency room. During a stroke, every minute counts.

At the hospital, a stroke team will assess your condition and treat your stroke with medicine, surgery, or another procedure. Recovery depends on the severity of the stroke and the speed of treatment. A rehabilitation plan may help you return to your previous activities.

SIGNS AND SYMPTOMS OF STROKE

The signs and symptoms of a stroke often occur quickly but can develop over hours or even days. This sometimes happens when a transient ischemic attack (TIA)—a blockage that breaks up before it damages the brain—turns into a stroke.

The type of symptoms depends on the type of stroke and the affected area of the brain. Signs of a TIA or stroke may include:

- sudden confusion, trouble speaking, or trouble understanding speech
- sudden numbness or weakness, especially on one side of the body
- sudden severe headache with no known cause
- sudden trouble seeing from one or both eyes
- sudden trouble walking, dizziness, or loss of balance or coordination

CAUSES AND RISK FACTORS OF STROKE

Strokes are caused by blocked blood flow to the brain (ischemic stroke) or sudden bleeding in the brain (hemorrhagic stroke). Many risk factors can be changed to help prevent a stroke or future strokes.

Ischemic Stroke

About 87 percent of strokes are ischemic. The blockage in the brain is usually caused by a piece of plaque or a blood clot. If the blockage occurs locally in the brain, it is called "thrombosis." If the blood clot travels from somewhere else in the body, it is called an "embolism." Ischemic strokes are classified based on where the blockage occurs in the brain and where an embolism develops in the body.

Plaque buildup on the inner walls of the arteries can lead to atherosclerosis, which hardens and narrows the arteries, limiting blood flow. Plaque can build up in any artery, including those in the brain and neck. Carotid artery disease occurs when plaque builds up in the carotid arteries in the neck that supply blood to the brain, which is a common cause of ischemic stroke.

If a blood clot breaks away from plaque buildup in a carotid artery in the neck, it can travel to an artery in the brain. The clot can block blood flow to part of the brain, causing brain tissue death.

When plaque builds up on the inner walls of the arteries, it can lead to a disease called "atherosclerosis." Plaque hardens and narrows the arteries, limiting blood flow to tissues and organs. Plaque can build up in any artery in the body, including arteries in the brain and neck.

Carotid artery disease occurs when plaque builds up in the carotid arteries in the neck that supply blood to the brain. It is a common cause of ischemic stroke. Blood clots leading to stroke can occur due to other heart and blood conditions, such as atrial fibrillation and sickle cell disease. Regular blood transfusions are the only treatment for undetected strokes (silent infarcts) in children with sickle cell disease.

Hemorrhagic Stroke

Sudden bleeding can cause a hemorrhagic stroke. This can happen when an artery in or on top of the brain breaks open, causing the brain to swell and raising pressure in the brain, which can damage brain cells. There are two types of hemorrhagic stroke: intracranial hemorrhage (bleeding within the skull) and subarachnoid hemorrhage (SAH; bleeding between the brain and the membrane that surrounds it).

Conditions that make blood vessels in the brain more likely to bleed include:

- **Aneurysm**. A balloon-like bulge in an artery that can stretch and burst.
- **Arteriovenous malformations (AVMs)**. Tangles of poorly formed arteries and veins that can break open in the brain.
- **High blood pressure (HBP)**. Puts pressure on the inside walls of the arteries, making them more likely to break open.

RISK FACTORS FOR STROKE

Several risk factors for stroke can be treated or controlled:

- smoking
- high blood pressure
- obesity
- physical inactivity
- poor diet

Other risk factors include:

- **Age**. The risk is higher for babies under one year and older adults.

- **Mental health**. Anxiety, depression, high stress levels, long work hours, and lack of social contact.
- **Family history and genetics**. A higher risk if a family member has had a stroke, particularly at a younger age.
- **Environment**. Living or working in areas with air pollution.
- **Medical conditions**. Sleep apnea, kidney disease, and migraine headaches.
- **Lifestyle habits**. Excessive alcohol consumption, sleeping too much, and using illegal drugs.
- **Race and ethnicity**. Higher occurrence in Black, Alaska Native, American Indian, and Hispanic adults.
- **Sex**. Younger men are more likely to have a stroke, but women have a higher lifetime risk. Women using birth control pills or hormone replacement therapy and those who have HBP during pregnancy are at higher risk.
- **Inflammatory conditions**. Viral infections, lupus, and rheumatoid arthritis (RA).

PREVENTION OF STROKE

Heart-healthy lifestyle changes can help recover from a stroke and may prevent another one:

- Quit smoking.
- Choose heart-healthy foods.
- Aim for a healthy weight.
- Manage stress.
- Get regular physical activity.
- Get enough good-quality sleep.

Strokes are a serious medical emergency requiring immediate attention. Recognizing the signs and symptoms, understanding the types and causes, and managing risk factors through lifestyle changes can significantly reduce the risk and effect of a stroke.[1]

[1] "Stroke," National Heart, Lung, and Blood Institute (NHLBI), May 26, 2023. Available online. URL: www.nhlbi.nih.gov/health/stroke. Accessed July 22, 2024.

Chapter 18 | **Smoking and the Immune System**

Smoking harms the immune system and can make the body less successful at fighting disease. The immune system protects the body from infection and disease, fighting everything from cold and flu viruses to serious conditions such as cancer.

Additionally, smoking is known to compromise the equilibrium, or balance, of the immune system. This increases the risk of several immune and autoimmune disorders, where the immune system mistakenly attacks the body's healthy cells and tissues. New evidence finds that smoking is a cause of rheumatoid arthritis (RA), an autoimmune disease in which the immune system attacks the joints and causes swelling and pain. People with RA have a harder time getting around and performing normal daily activities. Smoking also interferes with the effectiveness of certain treatments for RA.

CIGARETTE SMOKE AND DISEASE

Cigarette smoke contains more than 7,000 chemical compounds. Many of them can interfere with the immune system, allowing diseases to progress when the immune system is not working effectively. Diseases that can be worsened by smoking include:

- viral and bacterial infections, especially of the lungs (e.g., pneumonia, influenza, tuberculosis)
- periodontal or gum disease
- bacterial meningitis (a disease that attacks the protective membranes covering the brain and spinal cord)
- infections that occur after surgery
- rheumatoid arthritis
- Crohn's disease (a serious disease of the digestive system)
- cancer

People who want healthy lives should not smoke. Smokers lose both quality of life (QOL) and years of life. Smokers who want to quit can get help from their doctors. Free help is also available by calling 1-800-QUIT-NOW or visiting smokefree.gov or cdc.gov/tips.[1]

TIPS TO ENHANCE IMMUNITY

Our immune systems are complex and influenced by many factors. Vaccines, such as the flu vaccine, build immunity against specific diseases. Additional ways to strengthen your immune system include eating well, being physically active, maintaining a healthy weight, getting enough sleep, not smoking, and avoiding excessive alcohol use.

Quit Smoking

Smoking can make the body less successful at fighting disease. Smoking increases the risk of immune system problems, including RA.

Eat Well

Eating well means emphasizing plenty of fruits and vegetables, lean protein, whole grains, and fat-free or low-fat milk and milk products. Eating well also means limiting saturated fats, cholesterol, salt, and added sugars.

Eating well provides multiple nutrients that support optimal immune function. However, too much of some vitamins and minerals can be harmful. Talk to your health-care provider if you think you need nutritional supplements.

Be Physically Active

Regular physical activity helps you feel better, sleep better, and reduce anxiety. Combined with eating well, physical activity can help maintain a healthy weight.

[1] "Smoking and Overall Health," Centers for Disease Control and Prevention (CDC), May 28, 2016. Available online. URL: www.cdc.gov/tobacco/sgr/50th-anniversary/pdfs/fs_smoking_overall_health_508.pdf. Accessed April 23, 2024.

Following the physical activity recommendations for your age provides immediate and long-term benefits. For example, being physically active helps protect you from the flu. Emerging research also suggests that physical activity may benefit immunity.

Maintain a Healthy Weight

Excess weight can affect how your body functions. Obesity, defined as a body mass index (BMI) of 30 or more in adults, is linked to impaired immune functions. Obesity may also lower vaccine effectiveness for numerous diseases, including influenza, hepatitis B, and tetanus.

Safe ways to help maintain a healthy weight include reducing stress, eating healthy foods, getting enough sleep, and engaging in regular physical activity.

Get Enough Sleep

Scientific evidence is building that sleep loss can negatively affect different parts of the immune system, leading to various disorders. Ensure you get the recommended hours of sleep per day for your age.

Avoid Excessive Alcohol

Over time, excessive alcohol use can weaken the immune system.[2]

[2] "Healthy Habits: Enhancing Immunity," Centers for Disease Control and Prevention (CDC), December 19, 2023. Available online. URL: www.cdc.gov/healthy-weight-growth/about/enhancing-immunity.html. Accessed July 22, 2024.

Smoking and the Immune System

Chapter 19 | **Tobacco Use and Mental Health**

Chapter Contents

Section 19.1 | The Vicious Cycle of Smoking and Mental Health Disorders

SMOKING AND MENTAL HEALTH

A larger proportion of people diagnosed with mental disorders report cigarette smoking compared with people without mental disorders. Among U.S. adults in 2019, the percentage who reported past-month cigarette smoking was 1.8 times higher for those with any past-year mental illness than those without (28.2% versus 15.8%). Smoking rates are particularly high among people with serious mental illness, who demonstrate greater functional impairment. Estimates suggest that as many as 70–85 percent of people with schizophrenia and 50–70 percent of people with bipolar disorder smoke.

Rates of smoking among people with mental illness were highest for young adults, those with low levels of education, and those living below the poverty level. The 2005–2013 National Survey on Drug Use and Health (NSDUH) data indicated that smoking among adults without chronic conditions has declined significantly but remains higher among those reporting anxiety, depression, and substance use disorders. Similarly, a recent study based on the 2006–2019 NSDUH data showed higher smoking rates in adults with psychiatric disorders than in those without. Most importantly, smoking rates among adults with major depression and/or substance use disorder declined significantly during 2006–2019 in every examined age, sex, and racial and ethnic subgroup except for non-Hispanic American Indian or Alaska Native adults. These results suggest that tobacco cessation is achievable among adults with psychiatric disorders and tobacco use.

Smoking is believed to be more prevalent among people with depression and schizophrenia because nicotine may temporarily lessen the symptoms of these illnesses, such as poor concentration, low mood, and stress. However, smoking cessation has been linked with improved mental health, including reduced depression, anxiety, and stress, as well as enhanced mood and quality of life (QOL).

SMOKELESS TOBACCO AND SUBSTANCE USE

In addition to smoking, there is also a higher prevalence of smokeless tobacco use among individuals with anxiety or substance use disorders. Other research drawing on data from the National Epidemiologic Survey on Alcohol and Related Conditions (NESARC) found that all types of substance dependence were associated with nicotine dependence. Smoking is also highly prevalent among people in treatment for substance use disorders, with most studies finding rates between 65 and 85 percent among people in addiction treatment.

HIGH CIGARETTE CONSUMPTION IN MENTAL HEALTH DISORDERS

People who smoke and have a mental health disorder tend to smoke more cigarettes than those in the general population. The average number of cigarettes smoked during the past month was higher among those with a mental illness compared with those without one—331 versus 310 cigarettes. High cigarette consumption is a particular problem for people with serious mental illness. Although adults with both tobacco addiction and co-occurring mental disorders apart from substance use disorders comprised only 7.1 percent of the total U.S. population, they consumed 34.2 percent of all cigarettes smoked in the United States, according to data from the 2001 to 2002 NESARC.

HIGH PREVALENCE OF SMOKING AMONG PEOPLE WITH SCHIZOPHRENIA

Researchers are working to identify the brain circuits that contribute to the high prevalence of smoking among people with schizophrenia. Schizophrenia is associated with widespread reductions in functional connectivity between the dorsal anterior cingulate cortex and diverse parts of the limbic system. One report identified 15 circuits for which the reduction of functional connectivity correlated with the severity of nicotine addiction.

SMOKING RATES AMONG PEOPLE WITH MENTAL ILLNESS

People with substance use disorders and other mental illnesses do not quit smoking at the same rate as those in the general population. Survey responses from people who have smoked at some point during their lives indicated that fewer smokers with mental illness had quit compared to those without psychiatric disorders: 47.4 percent of lifetime smokers without mental illness smoked during the past month, compared with 66 percent of those with mental illness. A recent study found that among U.S. adults in 2019, the percentage who reported past-month cigarette smoking was higher among those with past-year major depressive episodes than those without (24.2% versus 17.6%) and among those with past-year substance (alcohol or drug) use disorders than those without (35.8% versus 16.8%).

RISK OF RELAPSE

Having a mental disorder at the time of cessation is a risk factor for relapse to smoking, even for those who have sustained abstinence for more than a year. Many smokers with mental illness want to quit for the same reasons cited by others (such as health and family), but they may be more vulnerable to relapse related to stress and other negative feelings.

EFFECT ON MORTALITY

The disparity in smoking prevalence is costing lives. A recent study found that tobacco-related diseases accounted for approximately 53 percent of deaths among people with schizophrenia, 48 percent among those with bipolar disorder, and 50 percent among those with depression.

MISCONCEPTIONS ABOUT SMOKING AND MENTAL ILLNESS

Since the 1980s, many providers have believed that people with schizophrenia smoke to obtain relief from symptoms such as poor concentration, low mood, and stress. But research is now showing that smoking is associated with worse behavioral and physical health outcomes in people with mental illness, and quitting smoking is showing clear benefits for this population. Comprehensive tobacco control programs and enhanced efforts to prevent and treat nicotine addiction among those with mental illness would reduce illness and deaths. Integrated treatment—concurrent therapy for mental illness and nicotine addiction—will likely have the best outcomes.

EFFECTIVE TREATMENTS

Smokers who receive mental health treatment have higher quit rates than those who do not. Moreover, evidence-based treatments that work in the general population are also effective for people with mental illness. For example, people with schizophrenia showed better quit rates with the medication bupropion compared with placebo and showed no worsening of psychiatric symptoms. A combination of the medication varenicline and behavioral support has shown promise for helping people with bipolar and major depressive disorders quit, with no worsening of psychiatric symptoms. A clinical trial found that a combination of varenicline and cognitive behavioral therapy (CBT) was more effective than CBT alone for helping people with serious mental illness stop smoking for a prolonged period—after one year of treatment and at six months after treatment ended.

Addressing the high prevalence of smoking among individuals with mental health disorders is crucial for improving both their mental and physical health. Comprehensive and integrated treatment approaches that simultaneously address mental illness and nicotine addiction have the potential to significantly reduce the burden of disease and mortality in this vulnerable population. By continuing to develop and implement evidence-based treatments and support systems, we can help individuals with mental health disorders achieve tobacco cessation, leading to enhanced QOL and overall well-being.[1]

Section 19.2 | **Anxiety Disorders and Smoking**

WHAT IS ANXIETY?

Anxiety is the feeling of being frightened, nervous, or panicky. Most people experience anxiety from time to time in difficult situations,

[1] "Do People with Mental Illness and Substance Use Disorders Use Tobacco More Often?" National Institute on Drug Abuse (NIDA), January 2018. Available online. URL: https://nida.nih.gov/publications/research-reports/tobacco-nicotine-e-cigarettes/do-people-mental-illness-substance-use-disorders-use-tobacco-more-often. Accessed July 22, 2024.

but it usually subsides when the situation ends. Anxiety becomes a problem when it is hard to control and affects day-to-day life. Excessive anxiety can also be a sign of an anxiety disorder—a common but serious mental illness. Anxiety disorders affect many adults in the United States, with women being more than twice as likely as men to develop an anxiety disorder in their lifetime.

People with anxiety disorders experience fear or dread about things that may happen now or in the future. They may also have some of the following physical symptoms:

- upset stomach
- weakness
- shortness of breath
- nausea
- rapid heart rate
- hot flashes
- dizziness

It is common for people with chronic anxiety to suffer from other conditions, such as depression, irritable bowel syndrome (IBS), chronic pain, and asthma.

HOW ARE SMOKING AND ANXIETY LINKED?

Some regular smokers believe smoking eases anxiety and report this as a reason they continue to smoke. However, this is because smoking relieves their nicotine withdrawal symptoms, and this relief is only temporary. Unless the underlying issues are addressed, anxiety is likely to return, perpetuating the cycle.

There are many smoke-free ways to handle stress and anxiety. It is important to explore these methods to find one or more that works for you.[1]

[1] Smokefree Women, "Anxiety and Smoking," U.S. Department of Health and Human Services (HHS), September 6, 2018. Available online. URL: https://women.smokefree.gov/live-healthier/care-for-your-mind/anxiety-smoking. Accessed April 23, 2024.

HOW NICOTINE CAN WORSEN ANXIETY SYMPTOMS

It is common to think that smoking is a way to calm your nerves and deal with feelings of anxiety. However, nicotine can actually cause anxiety symptoms or make them worse.

Nicotine and mood are connected. Researchers know that nicotine in cigarettes affects your brain, including your mood.

While some regular smokers believe smoking eases anxiety, this is due to the temporary relief of nicotine withdrawal symptoms. This relief is short-lived. Unless the root causes of anxiety are addressed, it is likely to return, and the cycle of smoking and anxiety will continue.

There are many smoke-free ways to handle stress and anxiety. Finding effective smoke-free strategies can help break the cycle of smoking and anxiety, leading to better mental and physical health.[2]

Section 19.3 | Understanding the Link between Smoking and Mental Health Conditions

DEPRESSION AND SMOKING

Smokers are more likely to experience depression than nonsmokers. It is important to recognize the signs of depression and understand how smoking can exacerbate these conditions.

What Is Depression?

Depression can affect anyone, but it is more common among smokers. Factors such as race, location, or income do not influence the likelihood of developing depression.

Common factors leading to depression include:

- feeling lots of stress
- going through a difficult life event

[2] Smokefree.gov, "Anxiety and Smoking," U.S. Department of Health and Human Services (HHS), June 7, 2017. Available online. URL: https://smokefree.gov/challenges-when-quitting/cravings-triggers/anxiety-smoking. Accessed April 23, 2024.

- experiencing a significant life change, even if planned
- having a medical problem
- taking medication known to cause depression
- using alcohol or drugs
- having blood relatives who have had depression

For some individuals, depression is situational, triggered by events such as divorce or the death of a loved one. For others, it may occur intermittently throughout their lives.

Signs of Depression

While everyone has down days, prolonged sadness could indicate depression. The differences between sadness and depression include:

- **Duration**. Depression is persistent, felt every day or most days, and lasts at least two weeks, often much longer.
- **Severity**. Depression interferes with daily life, hindering work, family duties, and activities.

Common signs of depression include:

- feeling sad all the time
- losing interest in activities once enjoyed
- being irritable, easily frustrated, or restless
- having trouble sleeping, whether falling asleep, staying asleep, or oversleeping
- changes in appetite
- difficulty concentrating
- feeling tired despite adequate sleep
- feeling worthless
- having thoughts of death or self-harm

The Link between Smoking and Depression

Smokers are more prone to depression, though the exact reason is unclear. Mood changes are common after quitting smoking, often as part of nicotine withdrawal. These changes usually improve within a week or two. If they persist, consult your doctor, as depression might be the cause.

While smoking may seem to alleviate depression temporarily, it ultimately causes more harm.

Seeking Help for Depression

Many people find relief through treatment, which can reduce symptoms and shorten the duration of depression. Treatment options include counseling and medication.

COUNSELING

Also known as "talk therapy" or "psychotherapy," counseling can be an effective part of depression treatment. It typically focuses on current thoughts, feelings, and issues. Counseling involves working with a therapist to improve coping strategies, change problematic behaviors, and find solutions.

MEDICATIONS

Antidepressants can help stabilize mood and improve coping abilities. These medications require a prescription and should be used according to your health-care provider's instructions. Do not stop taking antidepressants without consulting your provider.

Immediate Help for Depression

If you or someone you know is experiencing distress or suicidal thoughts, seek help immediately. Call or text 988 or chat online for 24-hour, free, confidential support from trained counselors.[1]

SCHIZOPHRENIA AND SMOKING

People with schizophrenia are more likely to smoke. Although smoking may provide short-term relief from symptoms, it soon leads to the stress of nicotine withdrawal.

---

[1] Smokefree Women, "Depression and Smoking," U.S. Department of Health and Human Services (HHS), September 6, 2018. Available online. URL: https://women.smokefree.gov/live-healthier/care-for-your-mind/depression-smoking. Accessed April 23, 2024.

Problems Linked to Smoking and Schizophrenia

Smoking can worsen several aspects of schizophrenia, including:

- increased likelihood of hospitalization and severe psychiatric symptoms
- need for higher medication doses
- impaired brain functions such as memory, problem-solving, attention, self-care, interpersonal relations, and work performance
- higher risk of suicidal thoughts or attempts
- greater likelihood of death from heart disease or cancer related to tobacco use
- significant financial cost

Health Benefits of Quitting Smoking

Quitting smoking does not worsen schizophrenia symptoms and offers numerous benefits such as:

- reduced risk of suicidal thoughts or attempts
- decreased likelihood of developing serious conditions such as COPD, heart disease, or having a stroke[2]

Section 19.4 | Posttraumatic Stress Disorder and Smoking in Veterans

Veterans with posttraumatic stress disorder (PTSD) are more likely to smoke than those without PTSD. Many individuals with PTSD use smoking to manage their mood, stress, and anxiety. Stress for veterans can be linked to deployment experiences or the challenges of adjusting to life after the military. While smoking might seem to alleviate stress temporarily, it can exacerbate PTSD and related symptoms over time.

---

[2] "Schizophrenia and Tobacco Use," U.S. Department of Veterans Affairs (VA), July 6, 2018. Available online. URL: www.mentalhealth.va.gov/quit-tobacco/docs/SchizophreniaandTobaccoUse_508.pdf. Accessed April 23, 2024.

PROBLEMS ASSOCIATED WITH SMOKING AND POSTTRAUMATIC STRESS DISORDER

Smoking can worsen various PTSD symptoms and overall health, leading to:

- increased feelings of anxiety, re-experiencing trauma, avoidance behaviors, and emotional numbness
- difficulty falling asleep and poor sleep quality
- complications with certain medications
- a higher risk of serious health conditions such as cancer, chronic obstructive pulmonary disease (COPD), stroke, and heart disease

BENEFITS OF QUITTING SMOKING FOR VETERANS WITH POSTTRAUMATIC STRESS DISORDER

Quitting smoking, although challenging, is achievable for veterans with PTSD and will not worsen PTSD symptoms. The U.S. Department of Veterans Affairs (VA) offers support to help veterans quit smoking. Benefits of quitting include:

- reduced anxiety and alleviation of some PTSD symptoms, especially over time
- improved mood and quality of life (QOL)
- enhanced effectiveness of medications for depression or anxiety
- lowered risk of health issues such as cancer, COPD, and cardiovascular problems

STEPS TO QUIT SMOKING

To begin your journey to quit smoking, consider the following resources and strategies:

- Call the VA's tobacco quitline at 1-855-QUIT-VET (1-855-784-8838) Monday–Friday, available in English and Spanish.
- Sign up for the VA's SmokefreeVET text messaging program by texting VET to 47848 (or VETesp to 47848 for Spanish) or visit smokefree.gov/VET.

- Consult your VA primary care provider or psychiatrist about tobacco cessation medications and counseling options.
- Visit publichealth.va.gov/smoking.[1]

Quitting tobacco is beneficial for both physical and mental health in the long term. Although it may seem like tobacco use helps alleviate stress, it often worsens PTSD symptoms, such as sleep difficulties. Contrary to the myth, quitting smoking does not exacerbate PTSD symptoms if proper support is received, especially during the initial weeks after quitting.[2]

Section 19.5 | Co-occurrence of Nicotine Addiction and Substance Use Disorders

UNDERSTANDING CO-OCCURRING DISORDERS

What Are Co-occurring Disorders?

People with substance use disorders (SUDs) are at particular risk for developing additional primary conditions or chronic diseases. The coexistence of both a mental illness and an SUD is known as a "co-occurring disorder" and is common among those undergoing treatment.

Individuals with mental illness are more likely to experience an SUD than those without a mental illness. According to the Substance Abuse and Mental Health Services Administration's (SAMHSA) 2022 National Survey on Drug Use and Health, approximately 21.5 million adults in the United States have a co-occurring disorder.

Combining medications for SUDs with anxiety treatment medications can have serious adverse effects. Common benzodiazepines include Xanax, Valium, and Klonopin, among others.

---

[1] "PTSD and Tobacco Use," U.S. Department of Veterans Affairs (VA), August 30, 2017. Available online. URL: www.mentalhealth.va.gov/quit-tobacco/docs/PTSDandTobaccoUse_508.pdf. Accessed April 23, 2024.

[2] "PTSD and Tobacco Use," U.S. Department of Veterans Affairs (VA), November 16, 2022. Available online. URL: https://news.va.gov/111012/ptsd-bytes-20-ptsd-and-tobacco-use. Accessed April 23, 2024.

Co-occurring disorders can include any combination of two or more SUDs and mental disorders identified in the *Diagnostic and Statistical Manual of Mental Disorders, Fifth Edition* (*DSM-5-TR*). No specific combinations of mental and substance use disorders are defined uniquely as co-occurring disorders.

Common Mental Disorders Associated with Substance Use Disorders

The most common mental disorders associated with SUDs include:

- anxiety and mood disorders
- schizophrenia
- bipolar disorder
- major depressive disorder
- conduct disorders
- posttraumatic stress disorder (PTSD)
- attention deficit hyperactivity disorder (ADHD)

Substance Misuse in Patients with Mental Disorders

Patients being treated for mental disorders often misuse the following types of substances:

- tobacco
- alcohol
- opioids
- stimulants
- marijuana
- hallucinogens
- prescription drugs[1]

THE RELATIONSHIP BETWEEN SUBSTANCE USE DISORDERS AND SMOKING

How Are Substance Use Disorders and Smoking Related?

Adults with an SUD are three to four times more likely to smoke than those without an SUD. In fact, 50 percent of deaths among

[1] "Co-occurring Disorders and Other Health Conditions," Substance Abuse and Mental Health Services Administration (SAMHSA), February 1, 2024. Available online. URL: www.samhsa.gov/medications-substance-use-disorders/medications-counseling-related-conditions/co-occurring-disorders. Accessed April 23, 2024.

people with an alcohol use disorder who smoke are due to tobacco-related diseases.

Health Problems Associated with Substance Use Disorders and Smoking

When you have an SUD and smoke, you have a significantly higher risk of developing health problems, including:

- greater chances of cancer of the mouth, throat, and esophagus when smoking and drinking alcohol
- increased cravings for nicotine can elevate drug cravings, jeopardizing recovery
- higher risk for serious health conditions such as various types of cancer, chronic obstructive pulmonary disease (COPD), heart disease, and breathing issues

Quitting Smoking during Substance Use Disorder Treatment

It is possible to quit smoking while undergoing SUD treatment, and many individuals desire to do so. With support such as counseling and medication, you have a good chance of success. Contrary to some beliefs, quitting smoking during treatment or early recovery is achievable and beneficial. Health improvements from quitting smoking include:

- reduced risk of cancer, particularly of the mouth, throat, and esophagus, for those with an alcohol use disorder
- improved chances of avoiding relapse into alcohol or drug use
- lowered risk of lung disease, heart disease, Alzheimer disease (AD), and other tobacco-related conditions

Quitting smoking can help reduce the desire to use other substances, aiding long-term recovery.[2]

[2] "Substance Use Disorders and Tobacco Use," U.S. Department of Veterans Affairs (VA), July 6, 2018. Available online. URL: www.mentalhealth.va.gov/quit-tobacco/docs/SUDandTobaccoUse_508.pdf. Accessed April 23, 2024.

Chapter 20 | Tobacco Use and Sleep

THE RELATIONSHIP BETWEEN TOBACCO USE AND SLEEP

How Are Tobacco Use and Sleep Related?

People who use tobacco are more than twice as likely to report insufficient sleep compared to nontobacco users. While tobacco users may claim that they use tobacco to manage sleep problems, studies show that smokers are more likely to experience daytime sleepiness than nonsmokers. Although the nicotine in tobacco products may help you feel more alert during the day, it can cause or worsen sleep difficulties.

Sleep Problems Associated with Tobacco Use

Research indicates that, compared to nontobacco users, tobacco users:

- spend more time in Stages 1 and 2 of sleep, leading to more fitful sleep
- spend less time in Stage 3 of sleep, the period of restful, restorative sleep
- have a higher risk for sleep-disordered breathing, such as snoring and obstructive sleep apnea (OSA)

Benefits of Quitting Tobacco for Sleep

While quitting tobacco can initially worsen sleep problems due to nicotine withdrawal, these issues will decrease over time, and your overall sleep quality will improve.

When you quit tobacco, you:

- may fall asleep faster, have less interrupted sleep, and experience longer total sleep time

- improve mood, functioning, and quality of life (QOL), all of which are associated with better sleep quality[1]

SMOKING AND SLEEP PROBLEMS IN ADOLESCENTS: A STUDY OF BLACK AND WHITE YOUTHS

The relationship between smoking and sleep difficulties is not well understood in adolescents, particularly across different race/ethnic groups. Past research suggests that the stimulant effects of nicotine contribute to poor sleep quality in adults. However, the direction of this relationship in adolescents remains unclear.

Study Overview

A national adolescent cohort study (N = 1,931) from 2009 to 2012 evaluated the longitudinal effects of sleeping difficulty and youth smoking among non-Hispanic white (NHW) and non-Hispanic Black (NHB) youths. Smoking in the past 30 days and sleeping difficulty were measured at each wave. The study assessed whether smoking predicts subsequent sleeping difficulty and vice versa, controlling for BMI, depressive symptoms, drinking, soda consumption, snoring or sleep apnea, parent education, and gender.

Study Results

The study found significant reciprocal and prospective relationships between smoking and sleeping difficulty. However, the strengths of these relationships differed by race/ethnicity:

- Prior sleep problems predicted future smoking more strongly for NHB youth than NHW youth (beta = 0.05 versus beta = 0.02).
- Past smoking predicted future sleeping difficulty more strongly for NHW youth than NHB youth (beta = 0.04 versus beta = 0.02).

---

[1] "Sleep and Tobacco Use," U.S. Department of Veterans Affairs (VA), December 2, 2019. Available online. URL: www.mentalhealth.va.gov/quit-tobacco/docs/VAM_TH-094_Sleep_and_Tobacco_Use_One_Pager_508.pdf. Accessed April 25, 2024.

Tobacco Use and Sleep

Reciprocal and prospective relationships exist between youth smoking and sleeping difficulty across race/ethnic groups. Further research is needed to understand this complicated relationship and to evaluate why these effects differ between NHW and NHB youths. If confirmed by future studies, improving sleep quality in youth may differentially reduce smoking among NHB individuals, thereby narrowing health disparities between these populations.[2]

[2] "Relationships between Smoking and Sleep Problems in Black and White Adolescents," National Institutes of Health (NIH), March 26, 2021. Available online. URL: https://researchfestival.nih.gov/2015/posters/relationships-between-smoking-and-sleep-problems-black-and-white. Accessed April 25, 2024.

Chapter 21 | Smoking and Reproductive Health Risks

Chapter Contents

Section 21.1 | Effect of Smoking on Fertility, Pregnancy, and Reproductive Health

HOW DOES SMOKING AFFECT FERTILITY, HORMONE PRODUCTION, AND CONCEPTION?

Smoking cigarettes can negatively affect fertility and make it harder to conceive. Research shows that:

- smoking can reduce fertility, making it difficult to conceive
- smoking may negatively affect hormone production
- smoking and exposure to tobacco smoke can harm the reproductive system
- smoking can damage the deoxyribonucleic acid (DNA) in sperm

If you or a loved one is trying to conceive and uses tobacco, learn about quitting smoking at this web page (www.fda.gov/tobacco-products/health-effects-tobacco-use/what-its-quit-smoking) and start on the path to a smoke-free life.

HOW DOES SMOKING DURING PREGNANCY AFFECT YOUR BABY'S FETAL DEVELOPMENT?

Smoking during pregnancy can lead to complications and negative health effects on the unborn child, including miscarriage and death. Smoking during pregnancy can increase the risk of:

- pregnancy complications such as preterm labor and delivery
- low birth weight
- underdeveloped lungs
- birth defects such as cleft lip and/or cleft palate
- sudden infant death syndrome (SIDS)

Additionally, the chemicals in cigarette smoke may increase the risk of ectopic pregnancy, where a fertilized egg grows outside the womb, often resulting in the death of the unborn child and, in some cases, the mother.

Smoking during pregnancy may also result in miscarriage. Nearly all tobacco products, including most electronic cigarettes (e-cigarettes), contain nicotine, which can cross the placenta and interfere with fetal and postnatal development.

If you are pregnant and interested in quitting smoking, consult with your health-care provider to discuss your reproductive health. Free resources for quitting while pregnant are available, including a supportive texting program.

CAN SMOKING PUT YOU AT RISK FOR CERVICAL CANCER?

Yes, smoking cigarettes can cause cervical cancer. This type of cancer occurs in the cervix, the lower, narrow end of the uterus that forms a canal between the uterus and vagina. Quitting smoking can reduce the risk of cervical cancer within a few years.

CAN SMOKING PUT YOU AT RISK FOR ERECTILE DYSFUNCTION?

Yes, smoking can increase the risk of erectile dysfunction, a condition where achieving or maintaining an erection firm enough for satisfactory sexual intercourse becomes difficult.

CAN SMOKING INCREASE YOUR LIKELIHOOD OF DYING FROM PROSTATE CANCER?

Yes, smoking can increase the likelihood of dying from prostate cancer. The prostate is a gland in the male reproductive system that produces a fluid-forming part of the semen. Prostate cancer begins in the prostate, and smokers with prostate cancer may have a higher mortality rate compared to nonsmokers with the disease.[1]

---

[1] "How Smoking Affects Reproductive Health," U.S. Food and Drug Administration (FDA), November 9, 2021. Available online. URL: www.fda.gov/tobacco-products/health-effects-tobacco-use/how-smoking-affects-reproductive-health. Accessed April 25, 2024.

Section 21.2 | Effect of Maternal Tobacco Use on Child Health

THE IMPORTANCE OF QUITTING SMOKING DURING PREGNANCY

Smoking is widely known to cause cancer and other major health problems, and smoking during pregnancy can lead to serious complications. These complications include premature birth, birth defects, and sudden infant death syndrome (SIDS). Even exposure to secondhand smoke can pose health risks for both mother and baby.

It is best to quit smoking before becoming pregnant. However, quitting at any stage of pregnancy can still provide significant health benefits for both mother and baby. There is no guarantee that a previous healthy pregnancy will be repeated if smoking continues during a subsequent pregnancy.

HOW SMOKING AFFECTS FERTILITY

Smoking can cause fertility issues for both men and women. Women who smoke often have more difficulty conceiving compared to nonsmokers. In men, smoking can damage sperm and contribute to erectile dysfunction (ED), making it harder to father a child.

HARMFUL EFFECTS OF SMOKING ON MOTHER AND BABY

- **Growth retardation**. Smoking can result in the baby being born too small, even after a full-term pregnancy, due to slowed growth before birth.
- **Premature birth**. Smoking increases the risk of preterm delivery, which can lead to various health problems.
- **Lung and brain development**. Smoking can damage the baby's developing lungs and brain, with effects lasting into childhood and adolescence.
- **Abnormal bleeding**. Smoking doubles the risk of abnormal bleeding during pregnancy and delivery, posing dangers to both mother and baby.
- **Birth defects**. Smoking raises the risk of birth defects such as cleft lip and cleft palate, leading to feeding difficulties and potential surgery.

- **Sudden infant death syndrome.** Babies exposed to cigarette smoke during and after pregnancy have a higher risk of SIDS.

RISKS OF PREMATURE BIRTH

Babies born prematurely (three weeks or more before the due date) miss crucial growth stages in the womb, increasing the risk of serious health problems or death. Premature babies may face:

- low birth weight
- feeding difficulties
- immediate and long-term breathing problems
- cerebral palsy
- developmental delays
- hearing or eyesight problems

Premature babies often require extended hospital stays.

BENEFITS OF QUITTING SMOKING

Quitting smoking at any point during pregnancy provides immediate and long-term benefits for both mother and baby:

- increased oxygen supply to the baby within one day
- improved growth for the baby
- reduced risk of premature birth
- increased energy and easier breathing for the mother
- decreased risk of heart disease, stroke, lung cancer, and other smoking-related diseases for the mother

SUPPORT FOR QUITTING DURING PREGNANCY

Many pregnant women who smoke want to quit but find it challenging. It is important to seek support to navigate the unique challenges of quitting smoking during pregnancy. Resources available include:

- Help Her Quit Smoking (https://women.smokefree.gov/your-relationships/ask-for-help)
- Pregnancy, Motherhood, and Smoking (https://women.smokefree.gov/pregnancy-motherhood)
- Smokefree Women (https://women.smokefree.gov)

STAYING SMOKEFREE FOR A HEALTHY CHILD

Avoiding exposure to tobacco smoke is crucial for a child's health. Benefits of a smoke-free environment for children include:

- fewer coughs and chest colds
- lower risk of bronchitis and pneumonia
- fewer ear infections
- reduced frequency of asthma attacks and wheezing problems[1]

Section 21.3 | Smoking and Pregnancy: Myths versus Facts

Quitting smoking at any point during your pregnancy is one of the best things you can do for your baby. Here are some common myths about quitting and pregnancy:

MYTH 1: I AM PREGNANT AND HAVE BEEN SMOKING, SO THERE IS NO POINT IN STOPPING NOW.

Fact. Quitting smoking at any stage of your pregnancy has health benefits for you and your baby. Even after just one day of not smoking, your baby will get more oxygen, helping the baby's lungs develop well. Quitting now also lowers your chances of having a baby with low birth weight.

MYTH 2: QUITTING SMOKING WILL BE TOO STRESSFUL ON MY BABY.

Fact. Quitting smoking does not put extra stress on your baby. It is one of the best things you can do for your health and your baby's health during pregnancy—and after the baby is born. By quitting smoking now, you will be protecting your infant from the dangers of secondhand smoke and reducing the risk of sudden infant death syndrome (SIDS).

[1] "Smoking, Pregnancy, and Babies," Centers for Disease Control and Prevention (CDC), October 13, 2023. Available online. URL: www.cdc.gov/tobacco/campaign/tips/diseases/pregnancy.html. Accessed April 25, 2024.

MYTH 3: SMOKING FEWER CIGARETTES IS OK!

Fact. There is no safe amount of smoking. Every puff of a cigarette releases harmful chemicals that reach your baby and affect your health, too.

MYTH 4: SMOKING RELAXES ME, AND BEING RELAXED IS BETTER FOR ME AND MY BABY.

Fact. Smoking may make you feel calmer temporarily, but it harms your body more than it helps. Smoking speeds up your heart rate, increases your blood pressure, and raises carbon monoxide levels in your bloodstream, reducing oxygen for your baby.

MYTH 5: THERE IS NOTHING WRONG WITH HAVING A SMALL BABY!

Fact. Smoking during pregnancy increases the chances of having a low birth weight baby. Babies with low birth weight are more likely to have serious health problems that can affect them now, throughout childhood, and into adulthood.

MYTH 6: THE ONLY WAY TO QUIT SMOKING IS COLD TURKEY!

Fact. Pregnant women have other ways to quit smoking besides going cold turkey, which is quitting without any preparation or counseling. Smokefree Women (https://women.smokefree.gov/quit-smoking-women/how-to-quit/prepare-to-quit) offers many resources that can help you quit. Try signing up for a text message program, such as SmokefreeMom. If you are having trouble quitting after trying different methods, be open with your doctor about your challenges and ask if medication may be right for you and your baby.

MYTH 7: I SMOKED DURING MY LAST PREGNANCY AND HAD A HEALTHY BABY, SO THIS NEXT BABY WILL BE HEALTHY, TOO.

Fact. Every time you smoke during pregnancy, you put your baby's health at risk. If you smoked and had a healthy pregnancy in the past, it does not mean your next one will be healthy, too.

MYTH 8: I SMOKE, SO I SHOULD NOT BREASTFEED MY BABY.

Fact. According to the American Academy of Pediatrics (AAP), mothers who smoke are encouraged to quit smoking but can still breastfeed their babies. Breast milk provides essential nutrients for healthy growth and development. Not smoking while breastfeeding, waiting to smoke until after breastfeeding, and keeping your home and car smoke-free are crucial to protecting your baby from nicotine and secondhand smoke.[1]

MYTH 9: E-CIGARETTES ARE SAFE TO USE DURING PREGNANCY.

Fact. E-cigarettes and other products containing nicotine are not safe to use during pregnancy. Nicotine is a health danger for a pregnant woman and her developing fetus, potentially damaging the developing brain and lungs. Additionally, some flavorings used in e-cigarettes may be harmful.

MYTH 10: E-CIGARETTES CAN HELP YOU QUIT SMOKING DURING PREGNANCY.

Fact. E-cigarettes are not currently approved by the Food and Drug Administration (FDA) to help people quit smoking. Individual, group, and telephone counseling have been found effective in helping people quit smoking. If you are pregnant and cannot quit smoking on your own or with counseling, discuss the risks and benefits of FDA-approved medications with your health-care provider. After your baby is born, you will have more options for FDA-approved quit-smoking medications.

Quitting smoking at any stage of pregnancy is one of the best decisions you can make for your and your baby's health. Dispelling myths about smoking and pregnancy can help you make informed choices. Seek support and resources to ensure a healthier future for you and your child.[2]

---

[1] Smokefree Women, "Myths: Smoking and Pregnancy," U.S. Department of Health and Human Services (HHS), September 7, 2018. Available online. URL: https://women.smokefree.gov/pregnancy-motherhood/quitting-while-pregnant/myths-about-smoking-pregnancy. Accessed April 25, 2024.

[2] "E-cigarettes and Pregnancy," Centers for Disease Control and Prevention (CDC), May 15, 2024. Available online. URL: www.cdc.gov/maternal-infant-health/pregnancy-substance-abuse/e-cigarettes.htm. Accessed July 22, 2024.

Section 21.4 | The Effects of Smoking on Urologic Health

TYPES OF UROLOGIC CANCERS ASSOCIATED WITH SMOKING

- Smoking triples your risk for bladder cancer and can cause other cancers of the urinary tract.
- The more cigarettes you smoke each day, the higher your risk for kidney cancer.
- Men with prostate cancer who smoke are at higher risk of death due to the disease compared to nonsmokers.
- Men who smoke are more likely to have their prostate cancer diagnosed at a more advanced stage.

OTHER UROLOGIC CONDITIONS AFFECTED BY SMOKING

Smoking can cause harmful chemicals to build up in the urine. If you smoke, you may:

- increase your risk for kidney stone disease
- experience worse symptoms if you have interstitial cystitis (painful bladder syndrome)
- increase your risk for stress urinary incontinence

CAN SMOKING CAUSE ERECTILE DYSFUNCTION?

Cigarette smoke alters the blood flow needed for an erection, and smoking interferes with the healthy function of blood vessels in erectile tissue.

BENEFITS OF QUITTING SMOKING FOR UROLOGIC HEALTH AND SEX LIFE

- You will decrease your chance of getting bladder or kidney cancer.
- If you have prostate cancer and quit smoking, your health prognosis improves.
- You will be less likely to experience ED. The earlier you stop smoking, the more likely you can reverse ED symptoms.
- You will improve your fertility and chance of starting a family.

The tobacco quitlines can double your chances of quitting compared with getting no support at all. Call to make your quit plan, get individual counseling, and develop strategies for preventing relapse. Free help is also available at 1-800-QUIT-NOW and at smokefree.gov and www.cdc.gov/tobacco/campaign/tips/index.html.[1]

[1] "Urologic Health and Tobacco Use," U.S. Department of Veterans Affairs (VA), January 4, 2024. Available online. URL: www.mentalhealth.va.gov/quit-tobacco/docs/UrologicHealthandTobaccoUse.pdf. Accessed July 22, 2024.

Chapter 22 | **Smoking and Other Specific Health Consequences**

Chapter Contents

Section 22.1 | Smoking and Its Effect on Eyesight

OVERVIEW OF SMOKING AND EYESIGHT

Smoking is as harmful to your eyes as it is to the rest of your body. If you smoke, you can develop serious eye conditions that can cause vision loss or blindness. Two of the greatest threats to your eyesight are macular degeneration and cataracts.

Macular degeneration, also called "age-related macular degeneration" (AMD), is an eye disease that affects central vision. You need central vision to see objects clearly and for common tasks such as reading, recognizing faces, and driving. There are two forms of AMD: dry AMD and wet AMD. Macular degeneration always begins in the dry form and sometimes progresses to the more advanced wet form, where vision loss can be very rapid if untreated.

Cataracts cause blurry vision that worsens over time. Without surgery, cataracts can lead to serious vision loss. The best way to protect your sight from damage linked to smoking is to quit or never start smoking.

SYMPTOMS OF EYE DISEASES RELATED TO SMOKING

You may think your eyes are fine, but the only way to know for sure is by getting a full eye exam. AMD often has no early symptoms, so an eye exam is the best way to spot this eye disease early. An eye specialist will place special drops in your eyes to widen your pupils. This offers a better view of the back of your eye, where a thin layer of tissue (the retina) changes light into signals that go to the brain. The macula is a small part of the retina that you need for sharp, central vision.

When symptoms of AMD do occur, they can include the following:

- blurred vision or a blurry spot in your central vision
- the need for more light to read or do other tasks
- straight lines that look wavy
- trouble recognizing faces

Eye injections are often the preferred treatment for wet AMD. Your doctor can inject a drug to stop the growth of these blood vessels and prevent further damage to your eyes. You may need injections on a regular basis to save your vision.

HOW DOES SMOKING AFFECT YOUR EYES?

Smoking causes changes in the eyes that can lead to vision loss. If you smoke:

- You are twice as likely to develop AMD compared with people who do not smoke.
- You are two to three times more likely to develop cataracts compared with people who do not smoke.

PREVENTING VISION LOSS RELATED TO SMOKING

If you smoke, stop. Quitting may lower your risk for both AMD and cataracts. If you already have AMD, quitting smoking may slow the disease. AMD tends to get worse over time. Quitting smoking is something within your control that may help save your sight. Other healthy habits may also help protect your eyes from cataracts and AMD:

- exercise regularly
- maintain normal blood pressure and cholesterol levels
- eat a healthy diet rich in green, leafy vegetables and fish
- wear sunglasses and a hat with a brim to protect your eyes from sunlight[1]

Section 22.2 | **Smoking and Buerger Disease**

WHAT IS BUERGER DISEASE?

Buerger disease, also known as "thromboangiitis obliterans," affects blood vessels in the body, most commonly in the arms and legs. The blood vessels swell, which can prevent blood flow and cause clots

[1] "Vision Loss, Blindness, and Smoking," Centers for Disease Control and Prevention (CDC), October 13, 2023. Available online. URL: www.cdc.gov/tobacco/campaign/tips/diseases/vision-loss-blindness.html. Accessed April 26, 2024.

to form. This can lead to pain, tissue damage, and even gangrene (the death or decay of body tissues). In some cases, amputation may be required.

The most common symptoms of Buerger disease are:

- fingers or toes that appear pale, red, or bluish
- cold hands or feet
- pain in the hands and feet that may feel like burning or tingling
- pain in the legs, ankles, or feet when walking, often located in the arch of the foot
- skin changes or small painful sores on the fingers or toes

HOW IS SMOKING RELATED TO BUERGER DISEASE?

The exact cause of Buerger disease is unknown; however, tobacco use is strongly linked to its development. Researchers believe that chemicals in tobacco may irritate the lining of the blood vessels, causing them to swell. Almost everyone diagnosed with Buerger disease smokes cigarettes or uses other forms of tobacco, such as cigars and chewing tobacco.

To prevent Buerger disease, avoid smoking cigarettes or using any other tobacco products.

HOW IS BUERGER DISEASE TREATED?

There is no cure for Buerger disease. The only way to keep the disease from worsening is to stop using all tobacco products. Medicines do not usually work well to treat the disease but can help control the symptoms. Surgery may help restore blood flow to some areas. In severe cases, it may be necessary to amputate the hand or foot if infection or widespread tissue death occurs.[1]

[1] "Smoking and Buerger's Disease," Centers for Disease Control and Prevention (CDC), October 13, 2023. Available online. URL: www.cdc.gov/tobacco/campaign/tips/diseases/buergers-disease.html. Accessed July 22, 2024.

Section 22.3 | Smoking and Diabetes

OVERVIEW OF DIABETES

Diabetes is a disease that causes blood sugar levels in the body to be too high, putting the body at risk for many serious health conditions. More than 25 million adults in the United States suffer from diabetes, and the disease is the seventh leading cause of death. It is also a growing health crisis around the world.

The 2014 Surgeon General's Report found that smoking is a cause of type 2 diabetes, also known as "adult-onset diabetes." Smokers have a greater risk of developing type 2 diabetes than nonsmokers. The risk increases with the number of cigarettes smoked per day.

HOW SMOKING CAUSES TYPE 2 DIABETES

Smoking increases inflammation in the body. Inflammation occurs when chemicals in cigarette smoke injure cells, causing swelling and interfering with proper cell function. Smoking also causes oxidative stress, a condition that occurs as chemicals from cigarette smoke combine with oxygen in the body, damaging cells. Evidence strongly suggests that both inflammation and oxidative stress are related to an increased risk of diabetes.

Evidence also shows that smoking is associated with a higher risk of abdominal obesity, or belly fat. Abdominal obesity is a known risk factor for diabetes because it encourages the production of cortisol, a hormone that increases blood sugar. Smokers tend to have higher concentrations of cortisol than nonsmokers.[1]

ANNUAL DEATHS FROM DIABETES CAUSED BY SMOKING

According to the American Diabetes Association (ADA), diabetes was listed as the underlying cause of death for over 87,000 people in 2019, making it the seventh leading cause of death in the United

[1] "Smoking and Diabetes," Centers for Disease Control and Prevention (CDC), May 31, 2016. Available online. URL: www.cdc.gov/tobacco/data_statistics/sgr/50th-anniversary/pdfs/fs_smoking_diabetes_508.pdf. Accessed April 26, 2024.

States. An estimated 9,000 people in the United States die each year from diabetes caused by cigarette smoking.[2]

EFFECTS OF SMOKING ON PEOPLE WITH DIABETES

Studies have confirmed that when people with type 2 diabetes are exposed to high levels of nicotine, insulin (the hormone that lowers blood sugar levels) is less effective. People with diabetes who smoke need larger doses of insulin to control their blood sugar.

Smokers with diabetes are more likely to have serious health problems, including:

- heart and kidney disease
- poor blood flow in the legs and feet that can lead to foot infections, ulcers, and possible amputation of toes or feet
- retinopathy (an eye disease that can cause blindness)
- peripheral neuropathy (damaged nerves in the arms and legs that cause numbness, pain, weakness, and poor coordination)

Although we do not know exactly which smokers will develop type 2 diabetes, we do know that all diabetic smokers should quit smoking or using any type of tobacco product immediately. The health benefits of quitting begin right away. People with diabetes who quit have better control of their blood sugar. Studies have shown that insulin can start to become more effective at lowering blood sugar levels eight weeks after a smoker quits.

People who want to quit smoking can get help from their doctors. Free help is also available at 1-800-QUIT-NOW and at smokefree.gov and www.cdc.gov/tobacco/campaign/tips/index.html.[3]

CAN QUITTING SMOKING REVERSE TYPE 2 DIABETES?

While quitting cannot reverse diabetes, it can make it easier to manage your diabetes. The sooner you quit smoking, the sooner

[2] "How Smoking Can Increase Risk for and Affect Diabetes," U.S. Food and Drug Administration (FDA), December 4, 2023. Available online. URL: www.fda.gov/tobacco-products/health-effects-tobacco-use/how-smoking-can-increase-risk-and-affect-diabetes#3. Accessed April 26, 2024.

[3] See footnote [1].

your body can start to heal. The health benefits for people with diabetes who stop smoking begin immediately.

Quitting smoking can:

- make your diabetes easier to control
- help your body use insulin better
- give you better control over your blood sugar levels
- help you recover from surgery faster

Insulin can become more effective at lowering blood sugar levels just eight weeks after you quit smoking.

Talk with your health-care provider about whether trying U.S. Food and Drug Administration (FDA)-approved nicotine replacement therapies (NRTs) to quit smoking is right for you. Your health-care provider can help you create a plan to quit that is best for your health and help you better manage your diabetes.[4]

Section 22.4 | The Effects of Smoking on the Digestive System

Smoking affects the entire body, increasing the risk of many life-threatening diseases, including lung cancer, emphysema, and heart disease. It also contributes to various cancers and diseases of the digestive system. About one-fifth of all adults smoke, and each year, at least 443,000 Americans die from diseases caused by cigarette smoking.

THE DIGESTIVE SYSTEM

The digestive system comprises the gastrointestinal (GI) tract and the liver, pancreas, and gallbladder. The GI tract is a series of hollow organs joined in a long, twisting tube from the mouth to the anus, including the mouth, esophagus, stomach, small intestine, large intestine (colon and rectum), and anus. The liver, pancreas, and

[4] See footnote [2].

gallbladder are solid organs of the digestive system. This system helps digest food, breaking it down into nutrients the body needs for energy, growth, and cell repair.

SMOKING AND CANCERS OF THE DIGESTIVE SYSTEM

Smoking increases the risk of cancers of the:

- mouth
- esophagus
- stomach
- pancreas

Research suggests smoking may also increase the risk of cancers of the:

- liver
- colon
- rectum

OTHER HARMFUL EFFECTS OF SMOKING ON THE DIGESTIVE SYSTEM

Smoking contributes to many common disorders of the digestive system, such as heartburn, gastroesophageal reflux disease (GERD), peptic ulcers, and some liver diseases. It increases the risk of Crohn's disease, colon polyps, and pancreatitis, and it may increase the risk of gallstones.

Smoking, Heartburn, and Gastroesophageal Reflux Disease

Smoking increases the risk of heartburn and GERD. Heartburn is a painful, burning feeling in the chest caused by reflux, or stomach contents flowing back into the esophagus. Smoking weakens the lower esophageal sphincter, allowing stomach contents to reflux into the esophagus, causing heartburn and possibly damaging the esophageal lining.

GERD is a persistent reflux occurring more than twice a week. Chronic GERD can lead to serious health problems such as bleeding ulcers, narrowing of the esophagus, and changes in esophageal cells that can lead to cancer.

Smoking and Peptic Ulcers

Smoking increases the risk of peptic ulcers and sores on the inside lining of the stomach or duodenum. It may also increase the risk of *Helicobacter pylori* infection, slow the healing of peptic ulcers, and increase the likelihood of recurrence. Smoking also increases the production of harmful substances such as pepsin and decreases protective factors such as blood flow and mucus secretion.

Smoking and Liver Disease

Smoking may worsen liver diseases such as primary biliary cirrhosis and nonalcoholic fatty liver disease (NAFLD). Liver diseases may progress to cirrhosis, where scar tissue replaces healthy liver tissue, impairing liver functions. Smoking harms the liver's ability to process medications, alcohol, and toxins, affecting the dose of medication needed to treat illnesses.

Smoking and Crohn's Disease

Current and former smokers have a higher risk of developing Crohn's disease, an inflammatory bowel disease (IBD) causing irritation in the GI tract. Smokers with Crohn's disease are more likely to have severe symptoms, need more medications, require surgery, and have symptoms recur after surgery.

Smoking and Colon Polyps

People who smoke are more likely to develop colon polyps, growths on the inside surface of the colon or rectum. Smokers' polyps are larger, more numerous, and more likely to recur.

Smoking and Pancreatitis

Smoking increases the risk of developing pancreatitis and inflammation of the pancreas. The pancreas secretes digestive enzymes that, when inflamed, attack its tissues.

Smoking and Gallstones

Some studies suggest smoking may increase the risk of developing gallstones, although research results are inconsistent. Gallstones are small, hard particles that can cause inflammation, infection, and abdominal pain.

REVERSING DAMAGE TO THE DIGESTIVE SYSTEM

Quitting smoking can reverse some effects of smoking on the digestive system. The balance between harmful and protective factors in the stomach and duodenum returns to normal within hours of quitting. The liver's ability to handle medications also improves. However, former smokers may still have a higher risk of some digestive diseases than those who never smoked.

By quitting smoking, you can improve your digestive health and reduce the risk of many associated diseases and conditions.[1]

Section 22.5 | **Smoking, Gum Disease, and Tooth Loss**

WHAT IS GUM DISEASE?

Gum (periodontal) disease is an infection of the gums that can affect the bone structure supporting your teeth. In severe cases, it can lead to tooth loss. Smoking is a significant cause of severe gum disease in the United States.

Gum disease starts with bacteria on your teeth that get under your gums. If the bacteria remain on your teeth for too long, layers of plaque (film) and tartar (hardened plaque) develop. This buildup leads to early gum disease, called "gingivitis."

When gum disease worsens, the gums can pull away from the teeth and form infected spaces. This severe gum disease is called "periodontitis." The bone and tissue that hold the teeth in place can break down, causing the teeth to loosen and potentially require extraction.

[1] "Smoking and the Digestive System," National Institute of Diabetes and Digestive and Kidney Diseases (NIDDK), March 15, 2013. Available online. URL: www.niddk.nih.gov/-/media/Files/Digestive-Diseases/Smoking_Digestive_System_508.pdf. Accessed April 26, 2024.

WARNING SIGNS AND SYMPTOMS OF GUM DISEASE

- red or swollen gums
- tender or bleeding gums
- painful chewing
- loose teeth
- sensitive teeth
- gums that have pulled away from your teeth

HOW IS SMOKING RELATED TO GUM DISEASE?

Smoking weakens your body's infection fighters (your immune system), making it harder to fight off a gum infection. Once you have gum damage, smoking also impedes your gums' ability to heal.

WHAT DOES THIS MEAN FOR YOU IF YOU ARE A SMOKER?

- You have twice the risk of gum disease compared to nonsmokers.
- The more cigarettes you smoke, the greater your risk of gum disease.
- The longer you smoke, the greater your risk of gum disease.
- Treatments for gum disease may not work as well for people who smoke.
- Tobacco use in any form—cigarettes, pipes, and smokeless (spit) tobacco—raises your risk of gum disease.

PREVENTING GUM DISEASE

You can help avoid gum disease with good dental habits:

- Brush your teeth twice a day.
- Floss often to remove plaque.
- See a dentist regularly for checkups and professional cleanings.
- Do not smoke. If you smoke, quit.

TREATING GUM DISEASE

Regular cleanings at your dentist's office and daily brushing and flossing can help treat early gum disease (gingivitis).

More severe gum disease may require:

- deep cleaning below the gum line
- prescription mouth rinse or medicine
- surgery to remove tartar deep under the gums
- surgery to help heal bone or gums lost to periodontitis. Your dentist may use small bits of bone to fill places where bone has been lost or move tissue from one place in your mouth to cover exposed tooth roots

If you smoke or use spit tobacco, quitting will help your gums heal after treatment.[1]

Section 22.6 | **Smoking in People with HIV**

Smoking is a serious health threat for everyone, but it is especially dangerous for people living with human immunodeficiency virus (HIV). Smoking raises the risk of heart disease, cancer, serious lung diseases, and infections such as pneumonia. People with HIV are more likely to develop these harmful consequences of smoking than those without HIV.

Quitting smoking can improve the quality of life (QOL) for people with HIV and reduce HIV-related symptoms. When you quit, your risk for many serious illnesses, including heart attacks and pneumonia, decreases.

WHAT IS HUMAN IMMUNODEFICIENCY VIRUS?

HIV stands for "human immunodeficiency virus." If not treated properly, it can lead to acquired immunodeficiency syndrome (AIDS). In the United States, HIV is mainly spread by having unprotected sex or sharing needles or other drug equipment with someone who has HIV.

[1] "Smoking, Gum Disease, and Tooth Loss," Centers for Disease Control and Prevention (CDC), October 13, 2023. Available online. URL: www.cdc.gov/tobacco/campaign/tips/diseases/periodontal-gum-disease.html. Accessed April 26, 2024.

Once you have HIV, you have it for life. Your body cannot eliminate HIV.

HIV harms your body's infection fighters—the cells of the immune system called "CD4 cells," or "T cells." Over time, HIV can destroy so many of these cells that your body cannot fight off infections and disease. When this happens, HIV leads to AIDS.

HOW IS SMOKING RELATED TO THE HUMAN IMMUNODEFICIENCY VIRUS?

Smoking causes one in every five deaths in the United States each year. About one in five Americans smokes cigarettes.

If you smoke and have HIV, you are more likely to get HIV-related infections, including:

- thrush (a mouth infection, also called "oral candidiasis")
- hairy leukoplakia (white mouth sores)
- bacterial pneumonia
- *Pneumocystis* pneumonia (PCP), a dangerous lung infection

Smoking when you have HIV also increases your risk of developing other serious illnesses compared to nonsmokers with HIV. These illnesses can cause disability or even lead to early death. They include:

- chronic obstructive pulmonary disease (COPD), a serious lung disease that causes severe breathing problems and includes emphysema and chronic bronchitis
- heart disease and stroke
- lung cancer, head and neck cancer, cervical cancer, and anal cancer

HOW CAN THE HUMAN IMMUNODEFICIENCY VIRUS BE PREVENTED?

Currently, there is no vaccine to prevent HIV infection and no cure for HIV infection. You can lower your risk of becoming infected with HIV or spreading the virus to others by taking the following steps:

- Get tested regularly for HIV.
- Practice abstinence (not having sex).
- Remain faithful to your spouse or partner.
- Consistently use male latex or female polyurethane condoms.
- Do not share needles or other drug injection equipment.
- Limit alcohol use and avoid drugs that affect your judgment.

HOW IS THE HUMAN IMMUNODEFICIENCY VIRUS TREATED?

Human immunodeficiency virus is treated with a combination of drugs called "antiretroviral therapy." These medicines are taken daily to prevent the virus from multiplying and destroying your body's infection fighters—the CD4 cells. This helps protect you from life-threatening illnesses, such as pneumonia and cancer.

Antiretroviral therapy cannot cure HIV, but it helps people with HIV live longer, healthier lives.

It is crucial to take your HIV medicines exactly as directed. If you do not, your CD4 count may decrease, and your viral load may increase. Not taking your medicines as directed can also make the HIV resistant, meaning the medicines will no longer be effective. Smoking may limit how well HIV medicines work to fight the virus.

Tell your doctor if your medicines are making you sick. They may be able to help you manage side effects and feel better. Do not stop taking your medicines without consulting your doctor.[1]

[1] "Smoking and HIV," Centers for Disease Control and Prevention (CDC), October 13, 2023. Available online. URL: www.cdc.gov/tobacco/campaign/tips/diseases/smoking-and-hiv.html. Accessed April 26, 2024.

Section 22.7 | Smoking and COVID-19

Coronavirus 2019 (COVID-19) has many people feeling stressed, alone, or worried about their health. If you are trying to stop smoking or stay smoke-free, this added stress can be challenging. However, not smoking (or using any tobacco products) is one of the best ways to protect and improve your health.

As a smoker, you or those who care about you may be worried about a connection between COVID-19 and smoking. Scientists are still learning about the disease, but we know that:

- being a current smoker increases your risk for severe illness from COVID-19
- smoking weakens the immune system, making it harder for your body to fight disease
- if you continue to smoke, you have a greater risk for respiratory infections such as pneumonia, colds, or flu
- COVID-19 affects many of the same organs as smoking. For those with heart or lung disease caused by smoking, there is an increased risk for severe illness from COVID-19

BENEFITS OF QUITTING SMOKING

Soon after you stop smoking, your body begins to heal. Within the first few weeks and months, your lungs start to work better, and your risk for a heart attack decreases. The longer you go without smoking, the more time your body has to recover. No matter how old you are or how long you have been smoking, quitting smoking improves your health and can add years to your life.

QUIT SMOKING RESOURCES

There are many free or low-cost resources to help you quit smoking. Start by creating a plan and trying different tools to see what works for you.

- **Create a personalized quit plan**. This helps guide you through the process.
- **Sign up for Smokefree TXT**. Receive daily messages with tips, strategies, and support.

- **Download a Smokefree app.** The quitSTART app (https://smokefree.gov/tools-tips/quitstart) can help you learn how to quit, manage cravings, and track your progress.
- **Visit Smokefree on social media.** Stay connected and grow your support network.
- **Talk to a quit coach.** Call 800-QUIT-NOW (800-784-8669) to be connected to your state's quitline. Trained counselors provide tips and tools for quitting and may help you get free or reduced-cost nicotine replacement therapy (NRT) medications. Or call the National Cancer Institute Quitline at 877-44U-QUIT (877-448-7848) Monday through Friday from 9:00 a.m. to 9:00 p.m. for help in English or Spanish.
- **Chat with a quit smoking counselor.** The National Cancer Institute's (NCI) LiveHelp service (https://livehelp.cancer.gov/app/chat/chat_launch) is available Monday through Friday, 9:00 a.m. to 9:00 p.m. Eastern time, also available in Spanish.
- **Visit Smokefree Women (https://women.smokefree.gov/pregnancy-motherhood/quitting-while-pregnant) for tips on quitting while pregnant.** Pregnant women are at higher risk for severe illness from COVID-19 and could have worse pregnancy outcomes, such as preterm birth, if they contract COVID-19. Protect yourself from illnesses during pregnancy whenever possible.

IT IS ALWAYS A GOOD TIME TO QUIT

There has never been a better time to quit smoking. If you slipped or have returned to smoking, recommit to living without cigarettes. Quitting is not easy, but there are things you can do to protect yourself and others during the COVID-19 pandemic:

- **Learn about nicotine withdrawal.** Common symptoms include irritability, poor sleep, difficulty concentrating, or increased appetite. Some people report cold or mild flu-like symptoms after quitting.

Call your doctor if you are concerned about symptoms associated with COVID-19.

- **Try quit-smoking medications**. Consider using one or more of the seven U.S. Food and Drug Administration (FDA)-approved prescription and over-the-counter (OTC) medications that can more than double your chances of quitting. Your doctor can recommend the best options for you.
- **Manage your stress and be kind to yourself**. The stress and anxiety caused by the COVID-19 pandemic can lead to a relapse. If you slip, do not be too hard on yourself.
- **Look out for signs of depression**. If you or someone you know is in distress or having suicidal thoughts, get help immediately. Call or text 988 or chat online (https://988lifeline.org) for 24-hour, free, and confidential support from trained counselors.
- **Learn about secondhand smoke**. Make smoke-free rules at home. Do not smoke in your home or car, and do not allow others to smoke there either. Ask smokers in your home to keep cigarettes and lighters out of sight and to shower or change clothes after smoking.
- **Focus on what you can control**. COVID-19 has created a lot of uncertainty. Try to focus on what you can control instead of worrying about the unknown. Practicing mindfulness may help you stay focused and manage urges to smoke.
- **Do not give up**. If you had a slip or started smoking again due to stress, set a new quit date and try again. It often takes multiple attempts to quit for good.

Taking steps to quit smoking can significantly improve your health and help protect you from severe illness related to COVID-19. Use the available resources and support systems to assist you on your journey to becoming smoke-free.[1]

[1] Smokefree.gov, "Smoking and COVID-19," U.S. Department of Health and Human Services (HHS), November 20, 2020. Available online. URL: https://smokefree.gov/quit-smoking/why-you-should-quit/smoking-and-covid19. Accessed April 29, 2024.

Section 22.8 | **Smoking and Chronic Pain**

THE LINK BETWEEN SMOKING AND CHRONIC PAIN

Do you find yourself using tobacco when you are in pain? You are not alone. Many people smoke to deal with chronic pain. Almost 100 million Americans live with chronic pain, and they tend to smoke about twice as much as the general population.

KEY FACTS ABOUT SMOKING AND PAIN

- Smokers are more likely to report that tobacco relieves pain. However, they also tend to have higher levels of pain.
- Tobacco is not effective for long-term pain relief. While chemicals in tobacco, such as nicotine, may have a temporary pain-relieving effect, the pain persists after smoking stops and is often exacerbated by withdrawal symptoms.
- Daily smokers experience higher levels of pain during the first 12–24 hours of smoking abstinence. Smokers with chronic pain often have lower confidence in their ability to quit and anticipate more severe nicotine withdrawal symptoms than smokers without chronic pain.[1]

HOW SMOKING AFFECTS PAIN IN YOUR BODY

People with chronic pain smoke about twice as much as the general population, likely due to two reasons:

1. Smoking can cause or worsen chronic pain conditions.
2. Some people smoke to try to control or distract themselves from their pain.

Smoking can make certain conditions more painful, including:

- back pain
- tooth and gum pain

[1] "The Connection between Pain and Smoking," U.S. Department of Veterans Affairs (VA), March 14, 2021. Available online. URL: www.myhealth.va.gov/mhv-portal-web/ss20180919-tobacco-and-pain. Accessed April 29, 2024.

- headaches
- fibromyalgia
- rheumatoid arthritis (RA)

Additionally, if you have been diagnosed with cancer and continue to smoke, you are likely to experience more pain than those who have never smoked or who have quit.

THE CYCLE OF SMOKING AND PAIN

Some people believe smoking helps them deal with their chronic pain, so when they feel the pain coming on, they reach for a cigarette. Chemicals in cigarettes may temporarily relieve pain, but once you are done smoking, the pain remains, and you may begin to experience nicotine withdrawal, which can make the pain worse.

BENEFITS OF QUITTING SMOKING ON PAIN REDUCTION

- If you have conditions such as back pain, severe headaches, or fibromyalgia, quitting smoking can help reduce the associated pain.
- If you have cancer and quit smoking, you may significantly reduce the pain associated with your cancer symptoms and treatment over time.[2]

STEPS TO QUIT SMOKING

Be honest with your health-care team about your interest in quitting tobacco. Using secure messaging to talk with your doctor or therapist can help. Patients with chronic pain are encouraged to use medications and counseling while attempting to quit smoking. Patients with chronic pain tend to be more nicotine-dependent and may find quitting more difficult. Correct dosing of tobacco cessation medications is crucial for these patients to quit successfully.[3]

---

[2] "Pain Management and Tobacco Use," U.S. Department of Veterans Affairs (VA), July 6, 2018. Available online. URL: www.mentalhealth.va.gov/quit-tobacco/docs/PainManagementandTobaccoUse.pdf. Accessed April 29, 2024.
[3] See footnote [1].

Part 3 | **Smoking Cessation Strategies**

Chapter 23 | **Understanding the Benefits of Quitting Smoking**

There are many great reasons to stop smoking. Understanding how smoking affects you and your loved ones and discovering the benefits of quitting can provide the motivation you need to become smoke-free. Reflect on why you want to quit and remind yourself of these reasons whenever you need extra encouragement.[1]

IMMEDIATE REWARDS

There is no safe amount of cigarette smoke. When you smoke, the chemicals in tobacco quickly reach your lungs with every inhale, and your blood carries these toxins to every organ in your body. However, after you quit, your body begins to heal within 20 minutes of your last cigarette. The nicotine leaves your body within three days. As your body starts to repair itself, you may feel worse before you feel better. Withdrawal can be challenging, but it is a sign that your body is healing.

LONG-TERM REWARDS

Quitting smoking can add years to your life. Smokers who quit before age 40 reduce their risk of dying prematurely from smoking-related diseases by about 90 percent. Those who quit by age 45–54 reduce their risk by about two-thirds. By quitting and

---

[1] Smokefree.gov, "Why You Should Quit," U.S. Department of Health and Human Services (HHS), June 5, 2016. Available online. URL: https://smokefree.gov/quit-smoking/why-you-should-quit. Accessed April 30, 2024.

staying smoke-free, you can take control of your health and significantly lower your risk of death from lung cancer and other diseases such as heart disease, stroke, chronic bronchitis, emphysema, and at least 13 other types of cancer. Additionally, you will protect your loved ones from dangerous secondhand smoke and set a positive example, showing them that a life without cigarettes is possible.[2]

HEALTH BENEFITS OF QUITTING

The health benefits of quitting smoking extend to most major parts of the body, from the brain to the DNA (deoxyribonucleic acid).

Brain

- **Broken addiction cycle.** Quitting smoking can rewire your brain and help break the cycle of addiction. The large number of nicotine receptors in your brain will return to normal levels after about a month of being smoke-free.

Head and Face

- **Sharp hearing.** Quitting smoking will help keep your hearing sharp.
- **Better vision.** Stopping smoking will improve your night vision and help preserve your overall vision.
- **Clean mouth.** After a few days without cigarettes, your smile will be brighter. Quitting smoking will keep your mouth healthy for years to come.
- **Clear skin.** Quitting smoking is better than any anti-aging lotion. It can help clear up blemishes and protect your skin from premature aging and wrinkling.

Heart

- **Decreased heart risks.** Smoking is a leading cause of heart attacks and heart disease. Quitting can lower

[2] Smokefree.gov, "Reasons to Quit," U.S. Department of Health and Human Services (HHS), August 9, 2018. Available online. URL: https://smokefree.gov/quit-smoking/why-you-should-quit/reasons-to-quit. Accessed April 30, 2024.

your blood pressure and heart rate almost immediately, reducing your risk of a heart attack within 24 hours.

- **Thin blood**. Quitting smoking makes your blood thinner and less likely to form dangerous clots. Your heart will have less work to do, as it can move blood around your body more easily.
- **Lower cholesterol**. Quitting smoking will lower the levels of cholesterol and fats circulating in your blood, slowing the buildup of new fatty deposits in your arteries.

Lungs

- **Stop lung damage**. Scarring of the lungs is irreversible. Quitting before permanent damage occurs is crucial. Within two weeks of quitting, you may find it easier to walk up the stairs because you are less short of breath.
- **Prevent emphysema**. There is no cure for emphysema, but quitting smoking before extensive damage occurs will help protect you from developing the disease.
- **Return of cilia**. Cilia, which help keep your lungs clear, start to regrow and regain normal function quickly after you quit smoking.

DNA

- **Lower cancer risk**. Quitting smoking prevents new DNA damage and can even help repair existing damage. This is the best way to lower your risk of cancer.

Stomach and Hormones

- **Smaller belly**. Quitting smoking reduces belly fat and lowers your risk of diabetes.
- **Normal estrogen levels**. For women, quitting smoking will gradually return estrogen levels to normal, improving the chances of a healthy pregnancy in the future.

Erectile Dysfunction

- **Sexual healing**. Quitting smoking lowers your chances of erectile dysfunction and improves your chances of a healthy sexual life.

Blood and the Immune System

- **Normal white blood cell count**. Quitting smoking helps your body heal from smoking-related injuries, eventually normalizing white blood cell counts.
- **Proper healing**. Improved blood flow to wounds helps nutrients, minerals, and oxygen reach wounds, promoting proper healing.
- **Stronger immune system**. Your immune system will become stronger, and you will be less likely to get sick once it is no longer exposed to tar and nicotine.

Muscles and Bones

- **Strong muscles**. Quitting smoking increases oxygen availability in your blood, making your muscles stronger and healthier.
- **Stronger bones**. Quitting smoking reduces your risk of fractures now and later in life, keeping your bones strong and healthy.

Quitting smoking offers numerous immediate and long-term health benefits, not only for yourself but also for your loved ones. By understanding the positive changes that occur after quitting, you can find the motivation needed to stay smoke-free. Your journey to better health begins with your decision to quit, and the rewards will be well worth the effort.[3]

---

[3] Smokefree.gov, "Benefits of Quitting," U.S. Department of Health and Human Services (HHS), January 27, 2024. Available online. URL: https://smokefree.gov/quit-smoking/why-you-should-quit/benefits-of-quitting. Accessed April 30, 2024.

Chapter 24 | Trends and Behaviors in Smoking Cessation

Tobacco use can lead to tobacco dependence and serious health problems. Quitting smoking greatly reduces the risk of developing smoking-related diseases. Tobacco and nicotine dependence often require repeated treatments, but there are helpful treatments and resources available for quitting.

Smokers can and do quit smoking for good. Since 2002, there have been more former smokers than current smokers.

U.S. ADULT SMOKING CESSATION BEHAVIORS

- Most adult cigarette smokers want to quit. In 2015, 68.0 percent of adult smokers (22.7 million) said that they wanted to quit smoking.
- More than half of adult cigarette smokers report having made a quit attempt in the past year. In 2018, 55.1 percent of adult smokers (21.5 million) said that they had made a quit attempt in the past year.
- Fewer than 1 in 10 adult cigarette smokers succeed in quitting each year. In 2018, 7.5 percent of adult smokers (2.9 million) successfully quit smoking in the past year.
- Four out of every nine adult cigarette smokers who saw a health professional during the past year did not receive advice to quit. In 2015, 57.2 percent of adult smokers (18.8 million) who had seen a health

professional in the past year reported receiving advice to quit.

- Even brief advice to quit (less than 3 minutes) from a physician improves cessation rates and is highly cost-effective.
- Less than one-third of adult cigarette smokers use cessation counseling or medications approved for cessation by the U.S. Food and Drug Administration (FDA) when trying to quit smoking. In 2015, 31.2 percent of adult smokers (7.6 million) reported using counseling or medication when trying to quit.
    - In 2015, 6.8 percent of adult smokers (1.7 million) reported using counseling.
    - In 2015, 29.0 percent of adult smokers (7.1 million) reported using medication.
    - In 2015, 4.7 percent of adult smokers (1.1 million) reported using both counseling and medication when trying to quit.
- More than three out of five adults who have ever smoked cigarettes have quit. In 2018, 61.7 percent of adult smokers (55.0 million adults) who ever smoked had quit.

U.S. YOUTH TOBACCO CESSATION BEHAVIORS

- About two-thirds of youth tobacco users report wanting to quit, and nearly two-thirds report trying to quit in the past year.
    - In 2021, 65.3 percent of youth (middle and high school students) who currently used tobacco products reported that they were seriously thinking about quitting the use of all tobacco products.
    - In 2021, 60.2 percent of youth who currently used tobacco products reported that they had stopped using all tobacco products for one day or longer in the past year because they were trying to quit.

Quitting smoking significantly reduces health risks and is achievable with the right support and resources. Both adults and youth demonstrate a strong desire to quit, highlighting the importance of accessible cessation treatments and consistent encouragement.[1]

[1] "Smoking Cessation: Fast Facts," Centers for Disease Control and Prevention (CDC), March 21, 2022. Available online. URL: www.cdc.gov/tobacco/data_statistics/fact_sheets/cessation/smoking-cessation-fast-facts/index.html. Accessed April 30, 2024.

Chapter 25 | **Creating a Personalized Quit Plan for Smoking Cessation**

Quitting smoking is hard, but preparation can greatly enhance your chances of success. Creating a personalized quit plan can help keep you focused, confident, and motivated. Quit plans combine various strategies to help you overcome challenges and improve your chances of quitting smoking for good. Follow these steps to create your own customized quit plan and keep it readily available during your effort to quit.

PICK A QUIT DATE

Choosing a quit date is a crucial first step. Many smokers choose a date within two weeks to quit smoking, which provides enough time to prepare. Avoid choosing a day when you know you will be busy, stressed, or tempted to smoke, such as a night out with friends or a busy workday.

- **Next step**. Circle your quit day on your calendar. Write it out somewhere you will see it every day to remind yourself of your decision to become smoke-free and give you time to prepare to quit.

LET LOVED ONES KNOW YOU ARE QUITTING

Quitting smoking is easier with support from important people in your life. Let them know ahead of your quit date that you are planning to quit and explain how they can help you. Different people need different kinds of support, so be sure to communicate your specific needs.

- **Next step**. Review tips on getting support to ensure you get the help you need.

REMOVE REMINDERS OF SMOKING

Getting rid of smoking reminders, such as cigarettes, matches, ashtrays, and lighters, can keep you on track during your effort to quit. It may also help to clean and freshen up your environment, such as your home, car, and workplace, to remove the smell of cigarettes, which can trigger cravings.

- **Next step**. Throw away all your cigarettes, matches, lighters, and ashtrays. Do not save one pack of cigarettes "just in case."

IDENTIFY YOUR REASONS TO QUIT SMOKING

Everyone has their own reasons for quitting smoking, whether it is to be healthier, save money, or protect loved ones. As you prepare to quit, consider your reasons and remind yourself of them daily.

- **Next step**. Make a list of all the reasons you want to quit smoking and keep it in a place where you can see it every day. Review your list whenever you feel the urge to smoke to stay motivated.

IDENTIFY YOUR SMOKING TRIGGERS

Certain activities, feelings, and people can trigger your urge to smoke. Anticipate these smoking triggers and develop ways to deal with them.

- **Next step**. Make a list of everything that makes you feel like smoking and write down one way to deal with or avoid each trigger. Keep this list nearby during your effort to quit.

DEVELOP COPING STRATEGIES

Nicotine withdrawal can be unpleasant, but developing strategies to cope with withdrawal can help ensure you stay smoke-free. Medications and behavior changes can help manage withdrawal symptoms.

- **Next step**. Ensure you have quit-smoking medications on hand before your quit date. Develop other quit-smoking strategies to use alongside medications. Remember that withdrawal symptoms, including cravings, will fade with each smoke-free day.

HAVE PLACES YOU CAN TURN TO FOR IMMEDIATE HELP

The first few weeks of quitting smoking are the hardest. Make sure you have quit-smoking support options available at all times, such as a quitline, support group, or a good friend.

- **Next step**. Plan on using multiple quit-smoking support options and keep them handy in case you need them. Consider these options:
  - **SmokefreeTXT**. A mobile text messaging service (https://smokefree.gov/smokefreetxt) for adults and young adults in the United States trying to quit smoking.
  - **Quitlines**. Call 1-800-QUIT-NOW (1-800-784-8669) to talk to a quit-smoking counselor.
  - **Quit smoking apps**. Mobile apps (https://smokefree.gov/tools-tips/apps) can help you prepare to quit, provide support, and track your progress.
  - **Support groups**. Check your local government's website for quit-smoking programs in your area.
  - **Friends and family**. Support from loved ones can make a big difference.
  - **Medications**. Have quit-smoking medications such as patches, gum, or lozenges on hand.

SET UP REWARDS FOR QUIT MILESTONES

Quitting smoking happens one minute, one hour, one day at a time. Reward yourself for reaching milestones such as being smoke-free for 24 hours, one week, and one month.

- **Next step**. Plan out your milestones ahead of time and set up a smoke-free reward for each one. Treat yourself to a nice dinner, a day at the movies, or any other smoke-free activity to celebrate your accomplishments.

Building a personalized quit plan is essential for a successful smoking cessation journey. By preparing in advance, removing triggers, and leveraging support systems, you can increase your chances of quitting for good. Remember, each step brings you closer to a healthier, smoke-free life.[1]

[1] Smokefree.gov, "Have You Built a Quit Plan?" U.S. Department of Health and Human Services (HHS), August 9, 2018. Available online. URL: https://smokefree.gov/learn-about-quit-plans. Accessed July 23, 2024

Chapter 26 | The Role of Support in Smoking Cessation

Quitting smoking is hard, but your support can be an important part of a loved one's smoking cessation experience. Not sure how to help? Want tips for being a more effective part of your quitter's support system? Understand what smokers go through when they quit and how you can be there for them throughout the process.

HOW MUCH SUPPORT SHOULD I GIVE SOMEONE QUITTING SMOKING?

Everyone who quits needs a different amount or type of support. Just ask them what kind of support they want and how much.

WHAT RESOURCES ARE AVAILABLE TO HELP SOMEONE QUIT SMOKING?

- **Online tips, tools, and support**. Suggest using the resources available on Smokefree.
- **SmokefreeTXT**. Sign up online (https://smokefree.gov/smokefreetxt) or text QUIT to 47848 to get 24/7 support sent right to your phone.
- **Smartphone apps**. Free apps (https://smokefree.gov/tools-tips/apps) help track cravings and understand smoking patterns.
- **Social media**. Visit Smokefree on social media (https://smokefree.gov/about-us/social) to grow a support network and stay connected.

- **Quitline experts.** Call the National Cancer Institute's Quitline at 1-877-44U-QUIT (1-877-448-7848) Monday through Friday from 9:00 a.m. to 9:00 p.m. or find your state's quitline by calling 1-800-QUIT-NOW (1-800-784-8669).
- **Counselor chat.** Get real-time help from the National Cancer Institute's LiveHelp online chat (https://livehelp.cancer.gov/app/chat/chat_launch).

HOW LONG DOES NICOTINE WITHDRAWAL USUALLY LAST?

For most people, the worst symptoms of withdrawal last a few days to a few weeks. Be extra mindful of the things that could trigger their urge to smoke during this time. Have a distraction or backup plan ready in case a craving hits.

WHAT IF MY FRIEND OR FAMILY MEMBER IS PREGNANT?

Many smokers feel strong pressure to quit smoking when they become pregnant and often want to quit. However, being pregnant does not make quitting easier. Pregnant women can experience withdrawal and cravings just like those who are not pregnant. Having a baby can be very stressful, and many women use smoking as a way to cope. Your support is crucial in helping someone quit and stay quit.

WHAT IF THE PERSON DOES NOT WANT TO QUIT SMOKING RIGHT NOW?

Quitting smoking is the best thing a person can do for their health, but the decision to quit must be their own. You cannot force them if they are not ready. However, continue to bring up the topic and let them know you will support them when they are ready.

WHAT IF I SMOKE?

If your friend or family member is quitting, and you have also been thinking about it, now could be a good time to quit. If you are not ready to quit smoking, decide how to handle your smoking around them to avoid triggering their urge to smoke. Consider the following:

- Do not smoke around them or buy cigarettes when you are together.
- Use mouthwash, wash your hands, and change your clothes to avoid smelling like cigarettes when you are together.
- Create a "no smoking" rule for your home and car if you live together.
- Keep your ashtrays, lighters, and cigarettes out of sight.
- Spend time in smoke-free places.

Supporting someone in their journey to quit smoking can make a significant difference in their success. By understanding their needs, providing the right resources, and offering consistent encouragement, you can help them overcome the challenges of quitting. Remember, your support is invaluable in helping them achieve a healthier, smoke-free life.[1]

[1] Smokefree.gov, "Help Others Quit," U.S. Department of Health and Human Services (HHS), June 18, 2024. Available online. URL: https://smokefree.gov/help-others-quit. Accessed July 23, 2024.

Chapter 27 | How to Quit Dipping or Chewing Tobacco

Quitting smokeless tobacco is challenging, but having a plan can help. Here are some tips for quitting chew and dip.

PICK A QUIT DATE

Every day is a good day to stop chewing tobacco or dipping. To prepare, try to pick a date within the next two weeks. A time with low stress works well for many people.

UNDERSTAND NICOTINE WITHDRAWAL

After you quit, you may feel uncomfortable and crave a chew or dip. This is withdrawal. Your body is getting used to not having nicotine. During withdrawal, you may:

- feel a little depressed
- be unable to sleep
- become cranky, frustrated, or mad
- feel anxious, nervous, or restless
- have trouble thinking clearly

The timeline for withdrawal symptoms can vary, but for most people, the worst symptoms last a few days to a few weeks. You may be tempted to chew or dip when these feelings hit. Remember that they are temporary, no matter how powerful they feel at the time.

LEARN HOW TO HANDLE TRIGGERS AND CRAVINGS

Triggers are specific people, places, or activities that make you want to chew or dip. Knowing your triggers can help you find ways to deal with them. Different people have different triggers. Some common ones are:

- waking up during the night or having nightmares
- after meals or during breaks
- driving
- stress or pain
- feeling anxious, angry, impatient, or bored
- seeing someone else smoke, chew, or dip
- drinking coffee or alcohol
- after sex
- before bedtime
- watching TV or a live game
- playing a sport

Triggers can cause cravings. Cravings are short but intense urges to chew or dip. All cravings are temporary and will pass with time.

TALK TO YOUR HEALTH-CARE PROVIDER

Talking with a health-care provider is a great first step in quitting tobacco. They will work with you to determine the treatment option that is best for you, including medications and counseling. Discuss with your provider the best type of nicotine replacement therapy (NRT) or other quit medication for you and the recommended dosage. Share the following information with them:

- medications and other quit methods you have used in the past and how you responded to them
- how much you currently smoke, dip, or chew
- any other medical conditions you have

This information will help you and your provider find a medication and quit plan that works for you and your life. Here are some questions to ask your provider when discussing medications:

- When do I start the medication?
- How long is the medication used for?

- How do I properly use the medication?
- What happens if I slip and use tobacco while taking this medication?
- What are the potential side effects? Is there anything I can do to minimize them?
- Is this medication right for me, given my medical history?

CELEBRATE SUCCESSES

An hour, a day, or any time without dipping or chewing tobacco is something to celebrate. Get together with the people who have supported your quit journey. Take time to feel proud of yourself.

BE PREPARED FOR THE UNIQUE CHALLENGES OF QUITTING

People who use smokeless tobacco face unique challenges when trying to quit. It is not the same as quitting cigarettes. There is more nicotine in smokeless tobacco, and the stressors can be different. Tailored resources can help make quitting chewing tobacco or dip easier.[1]

[1] Smokefree Veterans, "How to Quit Dipping or Chewing Tobacco," U.S. Department of Health and Human Services (HHS), July 8, 2024. Available online. URL: https://veterans.smokefree.gov/quit-dip-vapes/smokeless-tobacco/how-to-quit. Accessed July 23, 2024.

Chapter 28 | Quitting as a Woman

Chapter Contents

UNDERSTANDING UNIQUE CHALLENGES

Women can face different challenges when quitting smoking. Learning what makes quitting unique for some women can set you up for smoke-free success. Knowing what to expect can help you prepare to quit.

TRIGGERS

Negative emotions and reminders of smoking are powerful triggers for many smokers. Some women are very sensitive to these types of triggers. Feeling stressed or sad can make it harder to quit and stay quit. Seeing or smelling a cigarette can also make you want to smoke.

Learning how to handle difficult times without using cigarettes can help you avoid slips and stay smoke-free. Create an environment that supports your success by surrounding yourself with supportive people who want to help you become smoke-free.

WORRIES ABOUT WEIGHT GAIN

If you are worried about gaining weight after quitting, you are not alone. Many women who smoke have this concern. Focus on the benefits of quitting—such as improving how you look and feel. Becoming smoke-free can give you the confidence to reach other health goals. Do not let worries about weight gain stop you from trying to quit. Make becoming smoke-free your priority.

RELATIONSHIPS

Relationships are important in reaching smoke-free success, especially for women. Loved ones and partners can help you face challenges and celebrate milestones. However, being around people who are not supportive of your effort to quit can lead to slips or relapses. Planning ahead will help you manage situations with the people in your life while you try to quit.

- Identify people who will support your decision to quit and ask them for help.

- Take some time away (temporarily) from people who do not support your effort to quit.
- Buddy up with someone you are close with who smokes, and quit together. You will have a built-in support system and someone who understands the challenges of becoming smoke-free.

BEING A SMOKER

Many women worry that their life will change for the worse when they quit smoking. Some women who have quit return to smoking because they miss being a smoker. This might be because smoking and being a smoker has become an important part of their life, especially if they have been smoking for a long time. Thinking about why you smoke and what good things happen when you quit can help you mentally prepare to become smoke-free.

NICOTINE

Nicotine is the main addictive substance in cigarettes and other forms of tobacco. It affects many parts of your body, and up to 90 percent of people who smoke regularly are addicted to nicotine. Nicotine increases dopamine levels, a substance that makes the body feel good. When you stop smoking, your body has to get used to not having nicotine, a process called "withdrawal."

More research is needed, but women seem to have a slight advantage when it comes to nicotine addiction. When you smoke, dopamine is released, and because dopamine makes you feel good, you start to think of smoking as a reward. This seems to affect men who smoke more than women. It might be the reason women are more likely to smoke when dealing with stress or managing their moods, while men are more likely to smoke because of nicotine-related triggers such as craving and withdrawal. Learning ways to cope with stress and bad moods can help you avoid a slip or relapse after you quit.

QUITTING FOR TWO

Many women successfully quit smoking when they are pregnant or trying to have a baby. However, some women go back to smoking before or after their baby is born. The stresses of parenting and dealing with the changes in your life, relationships, and body can make it hard to quit before, during, or after pregnancy. Quitting smoking—at any time—gives you and your child important health benefits. Preparing to quit while pregnant and staying smoke-free after your baby is born will help you and your baby be happier and healthier.

QUIT ATTEMPTS

The unique challenges women face may contribute to why they typically try to quit more times than men before they quit for good. It might take you a few tries to become smoke-free, and that is okay. Each time you try, you learn what does and does not work for you, bringing you one step closer to a life without cigarettes.[1]

Section 28.2 | How Quitting Smoking Improves Women's Health

PHYSICAL BENEFITS OF QUITTING

Within 20 minutes of quitting, nicotine starts to leave your body, and it begins to heal. You will get some of these benefits right away. Quitting also improves your health in the years ahead and greatly reduces your risk of smoking-related illnesses. It is never too late to quit, no matter your age or how long you have been smoking. However, the earlier you quit, the better.

Healthier Blood, Heart, and Lungs

- **You will breathe easier**. Within two weeks of quitting, you might notice it is easier to walk up the stairs because you are less short of breath.
- **Your smoker's cough starts to go away**. You might cough more than usual when you first quit, but this is a sign that

[1] Smokefree Women, "How Quitting Can Be Different for Women," U.S. Department of Health and Human Services (HHS), September 6, 2018. Available online. URL: https://women.smokefree.gov/quit-smoking/what-women-should-know/how-quitting-is-different. Accessed May 2, 2024.

the cilia in your lungs are growing. They are among the first things in your body to heal after you quit.
- **Quitting can prevent permanent damage to your lungs.** Although scarring of the lungs is not reversible, quitting can prevent symptoms from getting worse if you have lung disease (such as chronic obstructive pulmonary disease (COPD)).
- **Normal oxygen levels aid heart function.** The oxygen in your blood rises to a normal level, making it easier for your heart to pump blood to important body parts.
- **Your heart rate and blood pressure lower, which puts less stress on your heart and lowers your risk of heart disease, including heart attacks.**

Stronger Body

- **Quitting can keep your bones strong and healthy, reducing the risk of fractures now and later in life.** This is important because both women and smokers are more likely than men and nonsmokers to get osteoporosis (a disease where your bones become weak and more likely to break).
- **Quitting can enhance immune system function.** Your immune system will become stronger, making you less likely to get sick.
- **Quitting can improve oxygenation and muscle health.** Quitting smoking will help increase oxygen availability in your blood, strengthening your muscles and making them healthier.

Changes You Can See

- **Your skin will look healthier.** Quitting can help clear up blemishes, protect your skin from premature aging and wrinkling, and help wounds heal better.
- **You will have a cleaner mouth.** Quitting will make your teeth brighter and gums healthier, and your breath will smell better.

- **Quitting can reduce belly fat and lower your risk of diabetes.** If you already have diabetes, quitting can help you manage your blood sugar levels.
- **Your sense of taste and smell will improve.** When you quit, you will taste foods better and smell foods, flowers, and other scents better.

Fewer Fertility Problems and Pregnancy Risks

- **Your estrogen levels will gradually return to normal.** Low estrogen can cause many problems, such as dry skin, thinning hair, and mood swings.
- **Quitting smoking will increase your chances of having a healthy pregnancy.** Women of childbearing age who quit smoking are less likely to have problems becoming pregnant. You will also lower your risk of certain pregnancy complications that can harm you and your baby, such as preeclampsia and placenta previa.
- **Quitting now will increase your chances of having a healthy baby.** Quitting at any time during your pregnancy lowers your risk of having a miscarriage. Quitting smoking also gives your baby benefits, such as lowering their risk of being born too early, having certain birth defects, or dying from sudden infant death syndrome (SIDS).

Long-Term Health Benefits

- **Heart disease.** Within 10–15 years of quitting smoking, your risk of heart disease may be the same as nonsmokers.
- **Stroke.** The longer you are smoke-free, the more your risk of stroke goes down. Within 5–15 years of quitting, your risk of stroke may be the same as nonsmokers.
- **Lung cancer.** The longer you are smoke-free, the more your risk of lung cancer goes down. Within 10 years of quitting, your risk of dying from lung cancer will have decreased by half.
- **Dying early.** People who smoke die about 10 years earlier than people who do not. Quitting can lower your risk of dying from smoking-related illnesses and diseases.

Benefits for Cancer Patients

If you have been diagnosed with cancer, it is not too late to benefit from quitting. Patients with some cancers increase their chances of survival if they quit when they are diagnosed with cancer. For those having surgery, chemotherapy, or other treatments, quitting smoking helps improve the body's ability to heal and respond to therapy. You will be less likely to develop pneumonia or respiratory failure. Quitting smoking may also reduce the chances that the cancer will recur (come back), that another cancer will develop, or that you will die from the cancer.

EMOTIONAL BENEFITS OF QUITTING

Quitting can improve your quality of life (QOL) and boost your mood. After you become smoke-free, you will experience many positive changes. Below are some things you may experience after quitting:

- You will feel more in control of your life. Being smoke-free means that you would not have to plan your life around smoking, worry about finding places to smoke, or worry about bothering others.
- Your hair, clothes, home, car, and breath would not smell like smoke anymore.
- You will have more money.
- You will have more energy to walk, play with your kids, or be active.
- Your loved ones will be proud of you.
- You will feel empowered and proud of your success.[1]

[1] Smokefree Women, "How Quitting Helps Women's Health," U.S. Department of Health and Human Services (HHS), September 6, 2018. Available online. URL: https://women.smokefree.gov/quit-smoking/what-women-should-know/how-quitting-helps-women. Accessed May 2, 2024.

Chapter 29 | **Behavioral and Technology-Based Treatments for Smoking Cessation**

Specialists in smoking cessation typically provide behavioral counseling for four to eight sessions. Both in-person and telephone counseling have been found beneficial for patients who are also using cessation medications. A variety of approaches to smoking cessation counseling are available.

COGNITIVE BEHAVIORAL THERAPY

Cognitive behavioral therapy (CBT) helps patients identify triggers—such as people, places, and things that spur smoking behavior—and teaches them relapse-prevention skills (e.g., relaxation techniques) and effective coping strategies to avoid smoking in stressful situations. A study comparing CBT and basic health education found that both interventions reduced nicotine dependence. However, another study found that among smokers trying to quit with the nicotine replacement therapy (NRT) patch, those who participated in six sessions of intensive group CBT had better-quit rates than those who received six sessions of general health education.

MOTIVATIONAL INTERVIEWING

In motivational interviewing (MI), counselors help patients explore and resolve their ambivalence about quitting smoking and enhance their motivation to make healthy changes. MI is patient-focused and nonconfrontational, and providers point out discrepancies between patients' goals or values and their current behaviors. They adjust to patients' resistance to change and support self-efficacy and optimism. Studies of MI suggest that this intervention results in higher quit rates than brief advice to stop smoking or usual care.

MINDFULNESS

In mindfulness-based smoking cessation treatments, patients learn to increase awareness of and detachment from sensations, thoughts, and cravings that may lead to relapse. This therapy involves patients purposefully attending to the thoughts that trigger cravings and cognitively reframing them as expected and tolerable. Patients learn techniques to tolerate negative emotions, including stress and cravings, without returning to tobacco use. Interest in mindfulness-based treatments has increased during the past decade, and studies show that this approach benefits overall mental health and can help prevent relapse to smoking. However, well-controlled clinical trials are needed.

TELEPHONE SUPPORT AND QUITLINES

As part of tobacco control efforts, all states offer toll-free telephone numbers (or quitlines) with smoking cessation counselors who provide information and support (800-QUIT-NOW or 800-784-8669). Studies of quitline interventions indicate that smokers who call quitlines benefit from these services, particularly when a counselor calls them back for multiple sessions. Although there is limited evidence on the optimal number of calls needed, smokers who participated in three or more calls had a greater likelihood of quitting than those who only received educational materials, brief advice, or pharmacotherapy alone. Quitlines have also been shown to help with smokeless tobacco cessation. The U.S. Department of Health and Human Services (HHS) provides a smoking quitline (877-44U-QUIT or 877-448-7848), as well as more information and tools for quitting (including text messages and other telephone-based support) at https://smokefree.gov.

TECHNOLOGY-BASED SUPPORT

Technology, including mobile phones, the Internet, and social media platforms, can be used to provide smoking cessation interventions. These technologies increase access to care by extending the work of counselors and overcoming geographical barriers that may deter people from entering treatment.

Text Messaging Support

Studies suggest that adults who receive encouragement, advice, and quitting tips via text message—a capability on even the most basic mobile devices—show improved quit rates compared with control programs. Text messaging provides an accessible and immediate form of support for those attempting to quit smoking.

Web-Based Services

Among adult tobacco users who called a "state quitline," most selected an integrated phone/web cessation program over a web-only intervention. Participants who chose the web-only option tended to be younger and healthier smokers with higher socio-economic status. These participants interacted intensely with the site once but did not re-engage as much as those who opted for the phone/web combination. A review of Internet-based smoking cessation programs for adults suggested that interactive Internet-based interventions tailored to individual needs can help people quit for six months or longer. Future research should determine the effectiveness of different technologies for smoking cessation support among populations that may be hard to reach, including those of low socioeconomic status and adults older than 50.

Social Media Support

Technology-based cessation interventions are particularly relevant to young adults aged 18–25, about 3.2 million of whom smoked daily in 2016. A systematic review and meta-analysis of published randomized trials of technology-based interventions—including computer programs, Internet, telephone, and text messaging—for smoking cessation among this population found that they increased abstinence by 1.5 times that of comparison subjects. Researchers recommend embedding cessation interventions in commonly used social networking platforms, and there has been some exploratory work in this area. Results of a trial with a relatively small number of participants suggested that Facebook was an accessible, low-cost platform for engaging young adults considering cessation. However, the study pointed to challenges in maintaining participation, retaining young people in the program, and the need for gender-specific features. A randomized controlled trial has been designed to test a stage-based smoking cessation intervention on Facebook tailored for smokers aged 18–25. Participants will be recruited online, randomly assigned to a Facebook group according to their readiness to quit, and will receive tailored daily messages and weekly counseling. The study will assess the intervention's influence on abstinence from smoking 3, 6, and 12 months after treatment, number of cigarettes smoked, quit attempts lasting 24 hours or more, and commitment to abstinence.[1]

[1] "What Are Treatments for Tobacco Dependence?" National Institute on Drug Abuse (NIDA), May 1, 2022. Available online. URL: https://nida.nih.gov/publications/research-reports/tobacco-nicotine-e-cigarettes/what-are-treatments-tobacco-dependence. Accessed May 2, 2024.

Chapter 30 | Nicotine Replacement Therapy

WHAT IS NICOTINE REPLACEMENT THERAPY?

Nicotine replacement therapy (NRT) is the most commonly used family of quit smoking medications. NRT reduces withdrawal feelings by giving you a small, controlled amount of nicotine without the other dangerous chemicals found in cigarettes. This small amount of nicotine helps satisfy your craving and reduces the urge to smoke.

Doctors and other medical experts consider NRT to be one of the most helpful tools for quitting smoking. Although some smokers experience mild to moderate side effects, research shows that NRT is safe and effective. NRT can be an important part of almost every smoker's quit strategy.

FORMS OF NICOTINE REPLACEMENT THERAPY

Nicotine replacement therapy comes in various forms, each used differently (see Table 30.1). You can choose the forms that work best for you. Some NRT products work better for certain people, so it might be worth trying different types to find what suits you best.

Table 30.1. Types of Nicotine Replacement Therapy

NRT Types	How to Get Them	How to Use Them
Patch	Over-the-counter	• Place on the skin. • Gives a small and steady amount of nicotine.
Gum	Over-the-counter	• Chew to release nicotine. • Chew until you get a tingling feeling, then place between cheek and gums.

Table 30.1. Continued

NRT Types	How to Get Them	How to Use Them
Lozenge	Over-the-counter	• Place in the mouth like hard candy. • Releases nicotine as it slowly dissolves in the mouth.
Inhaler	Prescription	• Cartridge attached to a mouthpiece. • Inhaling through the mouthpiece gives a specific amount of nicotine.
Nasal spray	Prescription	• Pump bottle containing nicotine. • Put into nose and spray.

NICOTINE REPLACEMENT THERAPY ALONG WITH OTHER STRATEGIES

Nicotine replacement therapy cannot do all the work. It can help with withdrawal and cravings, but it will not completely eliminate the urge to smoke. Even with NRT, quitting can be challenging. Combining NRT with other strategies can improve your chances of quitting and staying quit. A personalized quit plan can help you find tools and strategies that work together to keep you focused, confident, and motivated.

To give yourself the best chance for success, explore other quit methods you can combine with medication. Consider using:

- **Quit programs**. SmokefreeTXT (sign up online [https://smokefree.gov/tools-tips/text-programs/quit-for-good/smokefreetxt] or text QUIT to 47848).
- **Quitlines**. Call a quitline (https://smokefree.gov/tools-tips/get-extra-help/speak-to-an-expert) for additional support.
- **QuitSTART app**. Download the app (https://smokefree.gov/tools-tips/quitstart) for tips and inspiration to help you stay smoke-free.[1]

[1] Smokefree.gov, "Using Nicotine Replacement Therapy," U.S. Department of Health and Human Services (HHS), July 8, 2024. Available online. URL: https://smokefree.gov/tools-tips/how-to-quit/using-nicotine-replacement-therapy. Accessed July 23, 2024.

COMBINATION THERAPY

For some smokers, doctors may suggest using two NRTs or combining an NRT with a prescription medication. For example, a doctor may recommend combining a long-acting NRT like the patch with a short-acting NRT like nicotine gum to better control cravings.[2]

BUSTING NICOTINE REPLACEMENT THERAPY MYTHS

1. **Myth**. Nicotine replacement therapy does not work.
    - **Truth**. NRT can double a smoker's chances of quitting smoking for good. Many smokers find NRT helpful, and it may be worth trying to see if it works for you. Even if you have tried NRT before, it might be worth trying again, following directions carefully and using the recommended dosage and duration.
2. **Myth**. If I use NRT, I will not have withdrawal symptoms or cravings.
    - **Truth**. You may still have withdrawal symptoms or cravings while using NRT. Most people find withdrawal symptoms especially difficult in the first week or two after quitting. NRT can make these symptoms less intense. If withdrawal symptoms persist, talk to your doctor or pharmacist about different NRT products.
3. **Myth**. If I use one NRT product, I cannot use others.
    - **Truth**. NRT products can be used safely together. For example, you might use a long-acting NRT like the patch with a short-acting NRT like a lozenge. Combining products can help handle withdrawal symptoms and cravings.
4. **Myth**. Nicotine replacement therapy is too expensive.
    - **Truth**. Many states offer free NRT through state quitlines. People eligible for Medicare or Medicaid may also receive free NRT. Insurance coverage for NRT has

[2] Smokefree.gov, "Quit Smoking Medications," U.S. Department of Health and Human Services (HHS), July 8, 2024. Available online. URL: https://60plus.smokefree.gov/quit-smoking-60plus/quit-smoking-medications. Accessed July 23, 2024.

expanded under many private insurance plans. Even if NRT is not covered, its cost for several weeks is usually less than the cost of buying cigarettes.

5. **Myth**. Some people should not use NRT.
    - **Truth**. NRT is safe and effective for almost all adults. However, pregnant women, teens, and people with serious health issues should talk to their doctor before using NRT. Those with lung disease or heart problems may still use NRT but should seek medical advice first.[3]

[3] Smokefree.gov, "Busting NRT Myths," U.S. Department of Health and Human Services (HHS), July 8, 2024. Available online. URL: https://smokefree.gov/tools-tips/how-to-quit/busting-nrt-myths. Accessed July 23, 2024.

Chapter 31 | Effective Medications and Therapies for Quitting Smoking

Medications can make it easier to quit smoking by reducing cravings and withdrawal symptoms. Many former smokers find that using these medications for a couple of months helped them quit. However, they are just one type of tool, not a magic bullet. Follow instructions carefully to get the most benefit.

WHAT MEDICATIONS AND NICOTINE REPLACEMENT THERAPY PRODUCTS ARE AVAILABLE?

There are seven U.S. Food and Drug Administration (FDA)-approved medications: five nicotine replacement therapy (NRT) products (patch, lozenge, gum, nasal spray, and inhaler) and two prescription medications (Bupropion and Varenicline). Your pharmacist or doctor can help you choose which is best for you.

Nicotine Replacement Therapy

Nicotine replacement therapy works by giving you a small, controlled amount of nicotine, the main addictive substance in cigarettes and other tobacco products. NRT does not contain the other dangerous chemicals found in cigarettes. This small amount of nicotine helps satisfy cravings and reduces your urge to smoke. Some smokers experience mild to moderate side effects, but research shows that NRT is safe and effective. NRT is available over-the-counter (OTC) and by prescription.

Nonnicotine Prescription Medications

There are two common prescription medications that help smokers quit: Bupropion SR and Varenicline. You will need a prescription from your doctor to get these medications. Many insurance plans cover quit-smoking medications. Check with your insurance plan to see if you are covered.

BUPROPION SR

Bupropion SR (e.g., Wellbutrin) is a medicine without nicotine. It may help with withdrawal symptoms and the urge to smoke. This medicine may not be suitable for pregnant women, people with seizures, people with eating disorders, or heavy alcohol users.

VARENICLINE

Varenicline (e.g., Chantix) does not contain nicotine. This drug may help you quit by improving withdrawal symptoms and making nicotine from cigarettes less effective if you start smoking again. This medicine may not be suitable for people with kidney problems and women who are pregnant, planning to become pregnant, or breastfeeding.

Ask your doctor, dentist, or pharmacist if these medicines are right for you. Always use them as prescribed or as listed on the packaging.

Combination Therapy

For some smokers, doctors may suggest using two NRTs or combining an NRT with a prescription medication. For example, your doctor may recommend combining a long-acting NRT, like the patch, with a short-acting NRT, like nicotine gum, when you need extra help to control cravings.[1]

---

[1] Smokefree.gov, "Quit Smoking Medications," U.S. Department of Health and Human Services (HHS), June 18, 2024. Available online. URL: https://60plus.smokefree.gov/quit-smoking-60plus/quit-smoking-medications. Accessed July 8, 2024.

USING MORE THAN ONE MEDICINE CAN HELP A LOT

Nicotine patch plus lozenge or gum is the most common combination.

- How to use two NRTs together:
  - Put on a new patch each morning to get a steady level of nicotine that will reduce your cravings and withdrawal symptoms throughout the day.
  - Use a fast-acting nicotine medicine such as lozenges or gum to quickly combat cravings.
  - You can control how often you use the fast-acting medicine, so you will not get more nicotine than you want.

This combination is easy to use. Using two NRTs together can help you quit more successfully than using a single medicine.

ONE NONNICOTINE MEDICINE IS ESPECIALLY EFFECTIVE

Varenicline works to help people quit by attaching to the same parts of the brain that are stimulated by nicotine. This means that nicotine from a cigarette has fewer places to attach because the varenicline is already there. This makes it harder to get a nicotine "buzz."

- Varenicline:
  - reduces your urge to smoke and enjoyment of cigarettes
  - gives you the strongest chance for success of any single medicine
  - is started a week or more before you quit smoking

INCREASE YOUR CHANCES OF SUCCESS WITH QUIT-SMOKING MEDICINE

Get some free coaching to help you quit. Talking with a quit coach or a health-care professional such as your doctor or pharmacist will help you get the most out of the medicines you are using. You can also get other tips about ways to deal with urges to smoke. There are many ways to get help quitting:

- **Call 1-800-QUIT-NOW**. When you call a quitline, you will be connected to a quit coach who has been trained to provide you with the best quitting tips and tools, and to listen to and support you. Best of all, it is free, and sometimes quit coaches can help you get free quitting medications as well.

- **Talk with your doctor or other health-care professional**. Your doctor will be glad to hear you are interested in quitting. You can ask them for encouragement, suggestions, prescriptions if needed, and referrals to other support resources. They can also share with you how quitting smoking will dramatically benefit your health.
- **Check out free web, texting, and app programs**. Enrolling in a texting program (www.cdc.gov/tobacco/campaign/tips/quit-smoking/national-texting-portal.html), downloading an app (www.cdc.gov/tobacco/campaign/tips/quit-smoking/quitstart-app/index.html?s_cid=OSH_tips_D9871), or using a website designed to support quitting (https://smokefree.gov) can help you succeed. The web pages you are using now are another example. Many quitlines offer similar services.
- **Find a class or one-on-one counseling**. Group classes and one-on-one counseling may be available in your community and can help with quitting. You can check with your doctor or another health-care professional, your health insurer, or call 1-800-QUIT-NOW and ask about local resources.

GET QUIT-SMOKING MEDICINES FOR FREE OR REDUCED COST

- If you have health insurance:
    - Most health insurance plans cover FDA-approved quit-smoking medicines, including OTC medicines.
    - Even if you want to use an OTC medicine, you may need a prescription from your doctor for your insurer to cover it.
    - If you are unsure how to get them for free or at reduced cost, talk to your pharmacist or call the number on your insurance card. You can also call 1-800-QUIT-NOW, where a quit coach can help you connect with quit-smoking medicines.

- If you do not have health insurance:
  - Call 1-800-QUIT-NOW to ask about free or reduced-cost quit medicines.
  - Quit coaches can help connect you with quit-smoking medicines through community programs. Some states have special programs for people who smoke and do not have health insurance.
  - They may also be able to provide you with free medicines directly, such as by sending nicotine patches, lozenges, or gum to your home.
  - Try shopping around or using discount coupons. You may be able to buy nicotine patches, for example, for much less than the cost of a pack of cigarettes.
  - Look online or ask your pharmacist if they know about any discount programs you may be eligible for.
  - Once you quit, you will save the money you used to spend on cigarettes.

START TAKING SOME MEDICINES BEFORE YOU QUIT

It is okay to start nicotine patches, gum, or lozenges a week or two before you quit smoking. This can help you get ready and may cut down on your smoking. Starting medicine, especially the nicotine patch, before you quit may improve your chances of quitting successfully. If you start NRT while still smoking, it is important that you do so as part of an effort to quit completely, preferably in a week or two after starting the medicine.

Quit-smoking pills (varenicline or bupropion) are recommended to be started a week or more before quitting. Your doctor will discuss the best time to start when you get your prescription.[2]

[2] "Five New Ways to Quit with Medicines," Centers for Disease Control and Prevention (CDC), September 12, 2023. Available online. URL: www.cdc.gov/tobacco/campaign/tips/quit-smoking/quit-smoking-medications/5-new-ways-to-quit-with-medicines/index.html. Accessed July 8, 2024.

Chapter 32 | **Overcoming Challenges When Quitting**

Chapter Contents

Section 32.1 | Understanding and Managing Smoking Triggers

Triggers are the things that make you want to smoke. Different people have different triggers, such as a stressful situation, sipping coffee, going to a party, or smelling cigarette smoke.

Most triggers fall into one of these four categories:

- emotional
- pattern
- social
- withdrawal

Knowing your triggers and understanding the best way to deal with them is your first line of defense.

EMOTIONAL TRIGGERS

Many people smoke when they experience intense emotions. Emotional triggers remind you how you felt when you used smoking to enhance a good mood or escape a bad one. Examples include feeling:

- stressed
- anxious
- excited
- bored
- down
- happy
- lonely
- satisfied
- cooled off after a fight

Dealing with Emotional Triggers

- **Talk about your emotions**. Telling a friend or family member how you feel can help.
- **Take some slow, deep breaths**. Deep breathing will slow down your body, quiet your mind, and reduce cravings. It is also a great way to manage stress and anxiety.

- **Exercise**. Physical activity can help you handle emotions. When you exercise, your brain releases endorphins, chemicals that make you feel good.
- **Listen to calming music**. Music can relax you by slowing your heart rate, lowering blood pressure, and decreasing stress hormones.

PATTERN TRIGGERS

A pattern trigger is an activity that you connect with smoking. Examples include:

- talking on the phone
- drinking alcohol
- watching TV
- driving
- finishing a meal
- drinking coffee
- taking a work break
- after having sex
- before going to bed

Dealing with Pattern Triggers

- **Find a replacement**. Chew gum, eat sugar-free candy, or suck on a straw.
- **Try activities that keep your hands busy**. Squeeze a handball, do beading or needlework, or hold on to a coin or "worry stone."
- **Get moving**. Go for a walk, ride a bike, or go swimming. Exercising can distract you from smoking.
- **Change your routine**. For example, try drinking your coffee at a different time or brushing your teeth right after a meal.

SOCIAL TRIGGERS

Social triggers are occasions that usually involve other people who smoke. Examples include:

- going to a bar
- going to a party or other social event

- going to a concert
- seeing someone else smoke
- being with friends who smoke
- celebrating a big event

Dealing with Social Triggers

- **Avoid places where people smoke and ask your friends not to smoke around you.** Over time, it will get easier.
- **Tell your friends and family that you have quit and ask for their support.** They can help you avoid or cope with social situations that trigger your urge to smoke.

WITHDRAWAL TRIGGERS

Long-time smokers' bodies are used to getting regular doses of nicotine. When you quit, withdrawal symptoms will produce cravings for nicotine. Withdrawal triggers include:

- craving the taste of a cigarette
- smelling cigarette smoke
- handling cigarettes, lighters, and matches
- needing to do something with your hands or mouth
- feeling restless or having other withdrawal symptoms

Dealing with Withdrawal Triggers

- **Distract yourself.** Find something to take your mind off the craving.
- **Consider nicotine replacement therapy (NRT).** NRT can reduce withdrawal symptoms. Teens, pregnant women, and people with severe medical conditions should talk to their doctor before using NRT.

Now that you better understand triggers, identify the ones that you want to control, and make a plan to manage your cravings.[1]

---

[1] Smokefree.gov, "Know Your Triggers," U.S. Department of Health and Human Services (HHS), July 9, 2024. Available online. URL: https://smokefree.gov/challenges-when-quitting/cravings-triggers/know-your-triggers. Accessed July 11, 2024.

Section 32.2 | Effective Tactics for Handling Smoking Urges

DEALING WITH TRIGGERS AND CRAVINGS

It is no secret that quitting smoking is hard. You will not be able to avoid all your triggers, and learning how to deal with them takes practice. When a craving is triggered, it is important to have a plan to beat the urge to smoke.

Triggers lead to cravings to smoke. Cravings are uncomfortable, and the urge to smoke can be strong. The good news is that cravings are temporary, and there are things you can do to make yourself feel better during this time. Make a list of things to do when a craving hits. Here are some ideas:

- **Keep your mouth and hands busy**. Chew gum, suck on a straw, squeeze a handball, or do beading or needlework.
- **Exercise**. Go for a walk, ride a bike, or go swimming. Exercising can distract you from smoking.
- **Change your routine**. Try drinking your coffee at a different time or brushing your teeth right after eating.
- **Use nicotine replacement therapy (NRT)**. These medications can double your chances of quitting for good. Experiment with combinations of medications to see what works best for you.
- **Tell others that you are quitting**. Let the people in your life know you are quitting and ask them to avoid smoking around you. This will allow them to support you and might prevent them from offering you a cigarette.
- **Prepare to handle places where people smoke**. In the weeks or months after you quit, you might need to stay away from places where people smoke. The smell of cigarettes and other reminders of smoking can be a trigger, which might lead to a slip.
- **Take deep breaths**. Deep breathing can help your body relax by slowing down your body and reducing stress.
- **Let your feelings out**. Talk, laugh, cry, or write to express your negative feelings. It is okay to contact your family, friends, counselor, or loved ones for support.

It might take some time to find what works for you. Keep trying different things, and it will start to get easier.[1]

TIPS TO MANAGE URGES AND CRAVINGS

These strategies have been proven effective, with or without medications. You can try them when you decide to quit, or learn more by calling the free and confidential 1-800-QUIT-NOW quitline.

Adjust Your Medicine

If your urges are hard to resist, and you are using NRT, you may be able to use more. For instance, if you use a lower-dose patch, you can increase to a higher dose. Or you can add the nicotine mini-lozenge or gum. If you are using varenicline or bupropion, talk to your doctor or other health-care professional about your urges and these tips.

Make Your Environment Work for You, Not for Smoking

You can change some things about your home, car, and work to make it easier to quit and stay quit.

- Get rid of all cigarettes, lighters, matches, and ashtrays in your home, car, and at work before you quit.
- Wash your clothes and anything else that smells of tobacco smoke.
- Tell people you are quitting so they can support you.
- Avoid situations where you will be tempted to smoke, especially during the first few weeks.
- Tell friends who smoke that you are quitting and ask them not to smoke around you or offer you cigarettes.
- Ask the people you trust for help. Call a friend, go for a walk, or just talk to someone when you have an urge to smoke.
- Let your doctor and other health-care professionals know you are quitting so they can provide encouragement and additional suggestions.

[1] Smokefree Women, "Fight Cravings," U.S. Department of Health and Human Services (HHS), September 7, 2018. Available online. URL: https://women.smokefree.gov/quit-smoking-women/challenges-when-quitting/fight-cravings. Accessed July 7, 2024.

Watch Out for Other Temptations

- Be careful where you shop, especially at convenience stores where it is easy to buy cigarettes. Resolve before you go that you will not buy any cigarettes.
- Avoid places where smoking is allowed, especially during the first couple of months. Secondhand smoke and seeing others smoke can trigger cravings.
- Contact any tobacco companies that send you promotions or other mailings and request removal from their lists. You can also opt out of texts or emails from these companies.

Distract Yourself

When you have an urge to smoke, it may feel overwhelming. Distract yourself by focusing on something else:

- Listen to your favorite music.
- Go for a walk or do something physical.
- Call or text a friend.
- Play a video game or do a puzzle.
- Watch a funny video.

Practice these distractions before quitting to see what works best for you.

Find Safe Substitutes for Cigarettes

Keep substitutes for cigarettes handy when you quit. Some ideas include:

- Use toothpicks, straws, or cinnamon sticks to keep your mouth busy.
- Use paper clips, pencils for doodling, or a squeeze ball to keep your hands busy.

Practice using these substitutes before you quit to see which ones work best for you.

Listen to What the Urge Says, Then Talk Back!

Your thoughts may try to convince you to smoke, but you do not have to listen. Challenge these thoughts and talk back to them. For example:

- "I'm stressed, so I deserve a cigarette." Talk back by saying: "Yes, I'm stressed, so I deserve a break to breathe and relax."

- "If I don't smoke a cigarette right now, I'm going to go crazy." Talk back by saying: "This urge will pass, and once I quit for good, I'll feel less stressed."

Practice listening to urges and talking back before you quit.

Ride the Waves!

You do not have to give in to or fight your urges to smoke. Let the urge be, and it will go away on its own. Practice riding the wave of urges a few times a day before you quit. With time, your urges will weaken.

All of these tactics have been shown to help people quit smoking. They work best if you practice them before quitting.

Quitting smoking is challenging, but with a solid plan to manage triggers and cravings, you can increase your chances of success. Practice these strategies, use available resources, and stay committed to your goal of becoming smoke-free.[2]

Section 32.3 | Coping with Nicotine Withdrawal

When you stop smoking, your body needs to get used to not having nicotine. This can be uncomfortable, but there are ways you can manage nicotine withdrawal.

UNDERSTANDING WITHDRAWAL

Withdrawal is the collection of uncomfortable symptoms you have when you stop intaking nicotine. Nicotine is the main addictive drug in cigarettes and other tobacco products. For most smokers, the worst withdrawal symptoms last from a few days up to two weeks,

[2] "Tips for Quitting," Centers for Disease Control and Prevention (CDC), September 12, 2023. Available online. URL: www.cdc.gov/tobacco/campaign/tips/quit-smoking/tips-for-quitting/index.html. Accessed July 7, 2024.

but every smoker's withdrawal experience is different. Common withdrawal symptoms include:

- intense cravings for cigarettes
- feeling sad, irritable, or restless
- having trouble sleeping
- having trouble thinking clearly and concentrating
- feeling hungrier or gaining weight

WITHDRAWAL AND EMOTIONAL TRIGGERS

Negative feelings and mood changes can happen during withdrawal, and they can also be powerful smoking triggers. Learning how to manage emotional symptoms of withdrawal is very important to stay smoke-free. Try the tips below to help you get through it:

- **Build healthy coping skills**. Learn how to handle your emotional triggers without using cigarettes.
- **Consider using medication**. If you are not pregnant or trying to become pregnant, try nicotine replacement therapy (NRT) to help manage these symptoms and withdrawal-related cravings. You can also talk to your doctor about prescription medications that can help you quit.
- **Explore other ways to beat withdrawal**. The more tools you have at your disposal, the more successful you will be at dealing with triggers, cravings, and withdrawal.

GET SUPPORT

Having symptoms of withdrawal is a major challenge smokers face while quitting. Many people will start smoking again to feel better. There are ways to get support and avoid a slip or relapse:

- **Lean on your loved ones**. Let your friends and family know that quitting smoking may affect your mood and patience. Ask them to be understanding and supportive during this challenging time.
- **Connect with a trained quit-smoking counselor**. Call 1-800-QUIT-NOW (1-800-784-8669) or chat online at

LiveHelp (https://livehelp.cancer.gov/app/chat/chat_launch). Both services are available Monday through Friday, 9:00 a.m. to 9:00 p.m. EST.

WITHDRAWAL AND DEPRESSION

It is normal to go through negative mood changes after you quit smoking. This can be part of withdrawal. Some people feel sadder, irritable, or restless. However, if you feel very down for more than two weeks, it could be depression. If you think you have depression, try not to smoke. Talk to your doctor about your options for treating depression while staying smoke-free.

FIND HELP 24/7

If you or someone you know is in distress or having suicidal thoughts, get help now. Call or text 988 or chat online for 24-hour, free, and confidential support from trained counselors.[1]

Section 32.4 | Staying on Track with Your Quit Plan

Slipping and having a cigarette, or even going back to smoking for a little while, is not failing. It is a normal part of the quitting process. Get back on track and remember your goal to quit for good and your reasons for quitting. Understanding and preparing for the challenges you may face will help you become smoke-free.

Many people try quitting smoking multiple times before they finally succeed. Slips are a common part of quitting.

[1] Smokefree Women, "Dealing with Withdrawal," U.S. Department of Health and Human Services (HHS), September 7, 2018. Available online. URL: https://women.smokefree.gov/quit-smoking-women/challenges-when-quitting/withdrawal. Accessed July 23, 2024.

UNDERSTANDING SLIPS

A slip is one or two cigarettes after you quit. For most people, even "just one puff" counts. If you have a slip (having just one cigarette), it could be harder for you to stay smoke-free. But a slip is different from a relapse. A relapse means going back to smoking regularly.

You can learn from slips. Remind yourself that you have had a temporary setback. You have not failed, and you are not back to square one. A slip does not make you a smoker again. It also is not an excuse to relapse and go back to smoking regularly.

Prepare yourself to recover from slips and avoid a relapse. Think about how you will avoid or handle your triggers and deal with cravings.

SLIPS HAPPEN

Quitting smoking is a process that may take time. During that time, you might get frustrated. There is a chance you might slip at some point and smoke a cigarette. Slips happen to many people who quit smoking.

Slips often occur in the first three months after quitting, but they can happen any time. Many people need several tries before they quit for good.

It is possible to get back on track. Think about all you have accomplished. Stay positive and remind yourself that a slip is just one bump in the road on your smoke-free journey.

Knowing your triggers can help you understand what led to the slip. Find ways to avoid your triggers along the way. Having a plan to deal with cravings can help you get past them.

Use the quitSTART app (https://smokefree.gov/tools-tips/quit-start) to track your smoke-free progress, cravings, triggers, and smoking slips. You can tag the times and places that make it hard for you to stay smoke-free. The app will give you extra support when you need it most.

TIPS FOR MANAGING SLIPS

Many smokers slip and smoke a cigarette while they are quitting. You are not alone. Do not use a slip as an excuse to start smoking again.

If you slip, try these ways to get back on track:

- **Do not be too hard on yourself.** A slip does not make you a failure or mean you are relapsing. It does not mean you cannot quit for good.
- **Feel proud of the time you went without smoking.** Think about ways you avoided triggers and beat cravings. Try to use those strategies again.
- **Restart quitting right away.** Aim to restart today or tomorrow at the latest. Do not give up on your goal of no cigarettes at all.
- **Use a text message program.** If quitting forever seems too hard right now, try a program (https://smokefree.gov/tools-tips/text-programs/practice-quitting) to help you prepare to quit in the future. These programs help you build skills for dealing with cravings, triggers, and stressful situations. Try a Practice Quit (https://smokefree.gov/tools-tips/text-programs/practice-quitting/practice-quit) for a few days or a week of Daily Challenges (https://smokefree.gov/tools-tips/text-programs/practice-quitting/daily-challenges) without quitting. Sign up online (https://smokefree.gov/tools-tips/text-programs/practice-quitting) or by texting GO to 47848.
- **Use nicotine replacement therapy (NRT).** You do not need to stop using NRT after you slip and smoke one or two cigarettes. Using NRT increases your chances of staying smoke-free for good.
- **Get support.** If you slip, talk to family or friends. Ask them for help to stay smoke-free. You do not have to do it alone.
- **Reflect on what you learned.** Think about what helped you stay smoke-free and what caused you to slip. Consider what you can do differently to help yourself be smoke-free again.[2]

---

[2] Smokefree.gov, "Slips and Relapses," U.S. Department of Health and Human Services (HHS), June 18, 2024. Available online. URL: https://smokefree.gov/challenges-when-quitting/stick-with-it. Accessed July 23, 2024.

Section 32.5 | Overcoming Emotional Challenges Post-Smoking

MANAGING MOOD CHANGES AFTER QUITTING SMOKING

Mood changes are common after quitting smoking. You might feel irritable, restless, or down. If you experience these feelings after quitting, there are things you can do to help lift your mood.

Stay Active

Any kind of exercise can help—taking a walk, going to the gym, or joining a team sport. If needed, start small and build up over time. This can be hard when you're feeling down, but making the effort can pay off.

Structure Your Day

Create a plan to stay busy. Try to get out of the house whenever you can.

Do Things with Other People

Some people who are feeling down cut themselves off from others. Regular contact with people can help improve your mood. Try to connect with people regularly, whether in person, over the phone, or via text message.

Build Rewards into Your Life

For many people who feel sad, rewards and fun activities are missing from their lives. Finding ways to reward yourself can help lift your mood. Even small things, such as reading a magazine or listening to music, can add up and help you feel better.

Do What Used to Be Fun

One of the common signs of depression is losing interest in activities that used to be fun. It may be hard, but try doing enjoyable activities again to help improve your mood. Make a list of activities or events you enjoy and plan to do one each day.[1]

---

[1] Smokefree.gov, "Boost Your Mood," U.S. Department of Health and Human Services (HHS), June 18, 2024. Available online. URL: https://smokefree.gov/challenges-when-quitting/mood/boost-your-mood. Accessed July 23, 2024.

SEEKING SUPPORT AFTER QUITTING SMOKING

Ask for Help

You might like to solve problems on your own, but everyone can use a little help from time to time. If you are not sure how to ask, text a friend or send an email. You might say, "I want to quit smoking. Can you help?" Know an ex-smoker? Ask them why and how they quit.

Be Specific about What You Want

Your friends and family will not always know what help you need as you quit. Be specific about what support you want and do not want. Try to be nice about it. They are just trying to do what is best for you. For example, if you are feeling stressed after a long day at work and craving a cigarette, ask a friend to help plan a smoke-free night out to distract you.

Avoid Stressful Situations

Stress can make you feel like you want to smoke. Think about what stresses you most and look for ways to deal with that stress. Ask friends and family to be aware of your stressors. They can help make your life easier as you quit.

Say Thank You

Tell your friends you appreciate them, whether you speak it, text it, or show it with your actions. Saying thanks does not take a lot of time, so do it at the moment before you forget. Got a friend who gave up their last piece of gum to help you beat a cigarette craving? Buy some gum and give it to them with a note that says, "Thanks for helping me stay quit!" Studies show that being grateful can improve physical health, mental health, and self-esteem. Being grateful also can reduce stress.

Focus on People Who Can Help

If a friendship does not feel right anymore, it might be time to let it go. Do not be afraid to try a little distance with people who are not giving you the support you need. Letting go can be hard, but it is sometimes for the best. Focus on spending time with people who make you feel good about yourself and want you to succeed.

Invest in Your Relationships

The relationships you encourage and support the most may be the ones that are there for you the most while you quit. You will also feel more comfortable calling on them for support if the relationship is strong. You might go to a movie your friend really wants to see, even if it is not your top choice. Or go out of your way to call a friend just to chat and see how things are going.

Support Others

Support is a two-way street. If you want others to be there for you, you must be there for them, too. Check in with your friends and help them out when you can. Sometimes, small favors mean the most. Do something to brighten someone's day. Make a friend smile by emailing or texting them a joke, get someone a small treat for their birthday, or call a family member to see how they are doing. Do you have a quit method or quitting tip that worked for you? Post it on social media at SmokefreeUS (facebook.com/SmokefreeUS) or Smokefree Women (facebook.com/smokefree.women). Sharing your success can be a great motivator and support for others to become smoke-free.[2]

---

[2] Smokefree.gov, "Ask for Help," U.S. Department of Health and Human Services (HHS), June 18, 2024. Available online. URL: https://smokefree.gov/quit-smoking/getting-started/ask-for-help. Accessed July 23, 2024.

Chapter 33 | Lifestyle Changes after Quitting Smoking

Chapter Contents

Section 33.1 | Managing Appetite and Nutrition after Quitting Smoking

It is normal for your appetite to increase and your sense of taste to change after quitting smoking. By controlling your food choices, you can avoid overeating, weight gain, and poor nutrition. Increased appetite is a common withdrawal symptom that lasts longer than other symptoms. When you quit smoking, your senses of taste and smell improve, making food more enjoyable and potentially increasing your appetite.

SNACK SMART

When you quit smoking, you may miss the feeling of having something to do with your mouth and hands. Eating or snacking can mimic the action of smoking. This need to have something in your mouth will diminish over time. Keep your hands and mouth busy with a toothpick or straw, or chew on healthy foods such as carrots, celery, or sugar-free mints.

EAT MINDFULLY

People often use food the same way they used cigarettes—to deal with stress or boredom, reward themselves, pass time, or socialize. It is important to understand why you eat even when you are not hungry. Eat mindfully by eating slower and paying attention to your food. This can help you notice when you are full and enjoy your food more. Turn off the TV and put away your phone while eating to focus on the flavors and textures of your food.

CONTROL WEIGHT

Changes in your diet or eating more food might cause weight gain after you quit smoking. It is possible to manage your weight with a plan that addresses appetite and nutrition changes. Exercise can be a key part of this plan, helping you reduce cravings, appetite, and stress.[1]

SET HEALTHY EATING GOALS

You do not have to change your whole diet at once. Set reachable, positive, under-your-control, and specific goals. For example, "Cut up veggies and fruit in the evenings so I can take them in my lunch the next day," or "Eat a meatless dinner once a week, swapping veggies for the meat." Here are a few other goals that might work for you:

- Make half your plate a variety of different colored fruits and vegetables.
- Make half the grains you eat whole grains.
- Choose a variety of lean protein foods.
- Eat smaller portions.
- Drink water instead of sugary drinks.
- Eat some seafood every week.
- Prepare meals at home that consist of whole (unprocessed) foods.

Reward yourself when you reach each goal. Avoid using food as a reward. Treat yourself with extra time with a friend, a hobby you have wanted to try, or an activity that gets you moving. You can also combine rewards, such as taking a yoga class or going for a bike ride with a friend.

PLAN FOR HEALTHY MEALS

With a little planning, you can make dishes that are filling, healthy, and tasty. Think about your meals for the upcoming week and how much time you will have to make them. Go shopping with an ingredient list and try to stick with it. Pick items from the outer edges of the store, where they usually stock fresh and unprocessed foods.

[1] Smokefree.gov, "Nutrition and Appetite While Quitting," U.S. Department of Health and Human Services (HHS), June 18, 2024. Available online. URL: https://smokefree.gov/challenges-when-quitting/weight-gain-appetite/nutrition-appetite-while-quitting. Accessed July 11, 2024.

You can make healthier versions of your favorite dishes without losing the taste:

- Add spices and herbs instead of sauces.
- Bake or grill meat, poultry, or seafood.
- Roast veggies, meat, seafood, or poultry with a nonstick cooking spray or a small bit of olive oil.
- Sauté food using a nonstick vegetable spray, a small amount of broth, or a tiny bit of vegetable oil.

LEARN THE LABEL

When shopping, try to limit the amount of packaged foods you buy—they usually have hidden sodium (salt), saturated fats, or sugars. Even foods labeled "natural" or "healthy" can have hidden sugars under names like high-fructose corn syrup, barley malt, and dextrose. Before buying packaged food, check the Nutrition Facts label. It helps you know what is inside, manage portions, and stay healthy. Key parts of the Nutrition Facts label include:

- **Servings.** The label shows the serving size and the number of servings in the package.
- **Calories.** The label shows the calories per serving and sometimes per package. Calories measure the energy you get from a food serving. Eating too many calories per day is linked to overweight and obesity.
- **Ingredients.** The label lists several nutrients that can affect your health, with the most prevalent listed first.
- **% Daily Value (DV).** The % DV tells you the percentage of each nutrient in a single serving based on a 2,000-calorie diet. Your needs may vary.

SERVING SIZE AND PORTION CONTROL

A portion is the amount of food you choose to eat for a meal or snack. A serving is a measured amount of food or drink. Recognizing serving sizes can help control portion sizes and promote healthy eating. Try these tips:

- Measure out one cup, one-half cup, or one ounce of different foods into the plates, bowls, glasses, and cups you usually use.

- Eat meals on a smaller plate to reduce calorie intake while feeling satisfied.
- Measure single servings of your favorite snacks and store them in bags or containers.
- Wait 10 minutes before returning for seconds to see if you are still hungry. If you do go back, add veggies or fruit.
- At a restaurant, ask for a take-home container and put half your meal in it to save for later.

TRACK IT

Keeping a food diary can help you:

- Be aware of what, how much, when, and why you are eating.
- Eat mindfully by noting what you were doing or feeling at the time.
- Find where to make healthy changes, such as avoiding mindless munching.
- Identify overeating triggers, such as holidays or bad moods.

Consistently tracking what you eat is important. Do not be discouraged by occasional lapses. Your food diary is a tool for a healthier lifestyle now and in the future. You can even use free smartphone apps to help you track your eating habits.[2]

Section 33.2 | Staying Smoke-Free and Managing Weight Gain

Fear of gaining weight keeps some people from trying to quit smoking. When you make quitting your priority, it is the best step you can take for a healthier you.

[2] Smokefree Women, "Healthy Eating," U.S. Department of Health and Human Services (HHS), June 18, 2024. Available online. URL: https://women.smokefree.gov/live-healthier/care-for-your-body/healthy-eating. Accessed July 11, 2024.

SMOKING AND WEIGHT

It is true that some people gain weight after quitting. On average, people who gain weight after quitting gain about 5–10 pounds. Here is why:

- **Smoking lowers your appetite.** Smoking cigarettes makes you feel less hungry. When you quit smoking, you might feel hungrier and eat more.
- **Eating as a substitute for smoking.** Smoking gives you something to do with your hands, and you get used to putting a cigarette in your mouth. For many, food replaces cigarettes, leading to weight gain.
- **Eating to deal with negative emotions.** Smoking might have been your go-to when you felt stressed. When you quit, you may eat to feel better or to deal with stress, which can cause weight gain.

If you are worried about gaining weight after you quit, remember:

- Quitting smoking is the best thing you can do for your health right now.
- You can take steps to prevent weight gain while becoming smoke-free, such as healthy snacking, watching portion sizes, and finding 10 minutes a few times a day to move more.
- If you gain weight after quitting, it does not have to be permanent. There are healthy ways to lose weight.

SET REALISTIC GOALS

When trying to lose weight, think of steps that are manageable, positive, under your control, and specific. Every step toward your goal is a step to a healthier you. If your current plan is not working, change it. It may take a few tries to find what works best for quitting smoking and making other healthy lifestyle choices is no different.

HEALTHY WEIGHT LOSS AND BODY IMAGE

Becoming and staying smoke-free will give you more energy and confidence, which will help you lose any weight you might have gained after quitting. There is no magic number for healthy weight. Everyone is different. Trying to lose weight with extreme diets or over-the-top workouts does not work long-term. The key is slow and steady weight loss. Find what works for you and recognize your successes. Celebrate milestones such as losing 5 percent of your body weight, fitting into a pair of jeans that used to be too tight, or improving your jogging pace.

If weight gain is a big concern, think about why. Many people struggle with poor body image and unrealistic expectations of how they should look. Our bodies are capable of amazing things, and the better we treat them, the more they can do. Be easier on yourself and find things to love about your body.[1]

HOW TO CONTROL WEIGHT GAIN AFTER QUITTING

Control Your Appetite

Smoking cigarettes makes you feel less hungry. When you quit smoking, you might feel hungrier and eat more than you used to. Portion control can help you prevent overeating. Stay hydrated to avoid eating when you are actually thirsty.

Start Exercising Regularly

Smoking cigarettes increases your metabolism, so you burn more calories. When you stop smoking, you may burn fewer calories, which can lead to weight gain. Regular exercise can help you continue to burn those calories. Just 10 minutes of exercise a day can make a difference.

Learn How to Eat Mindfully

Eating can become a substitute for smoking. It does not have to. Learn how to eat mindfully. Mindful eating means preparing, choosing, and eating with awareness. Here are some tips to help you eat healthier and enjoy your food more:

- **Avoid distractions**. Turn off the phone, television, and computer.

[1] Smokefree Women, "Weight Gain and Quitting," U.S. Department of Health and Human Services (HHS), June 18, 2024. Available online. URL: https://women.smokefree.gov/quit-smoking-women/challenges-when-quitting/weight-gain. Accessed July 11, 2024.

- **Eat at your dinner table.** It helps to focus on what you are eating.
- **Think carefully about your portion sizes.** Consider starting with a smaller portion.
- **Avoid serving food family style.** If you still feel hungry, you will have to get up from the table for seconds.
- **Do a belly check.** Are you starving or eating for some other reason?

Learn to Cope with Emotions without Cigarettes

When you stop smoking, you may want to turn to eating when you feel bad or life is stressful. But you can learn other ways to cope without smoking, such as practicing relaxation techniques, taking care of yourself, and sharing your feelings with friends and family.[2]

Section 33.3 | **Physical Activity for Smoking Cessation**

MANAGING CRAVINGS WITH EXERCISE

Having cravings for a cigarette is one of the most common symptoms of nicotine withdrawal when you quit smoking. It helps to have a plan to manage cravings when they hit. Including exercise in your plan can help you get past cravings.

Exercise can distract you and keep you busy until the craving passes. Exercise has other benefits too:

- **Short periods of physical activity.** Studies show that even short periods of physical activity, especially aerobic exercise, reduce the urge to smoke. Aerobic exercise makes you sweat, causes you to breathe harder, and gets your heart beating faster. It strengthens your heart and lungs. Walking, swimming, running,

[2] Smokefree.gov, "Manage Weight Gain after Quitting," U.S. Department of Health and Human Services (HHS), June 18, 2024. Available online. URL: https://smokefree.gov/challenges-when-quitting/weight-gain-appetite/manage-weight-gain. Accessed July 11, 2024.

dancing, cycling, and boxing are a few types of aerobic exercise.

- **Reduced withdrawal symptoms and cravings.** Withdrawal symptoms and cravings for cigarettes decrease during exercise and up to 50 minutes after exercising.
- **Decreased appetite and limited weight gain.** Exercise decreases appetite and helps limit the weight gain some people experience when they quit smoking.
- **Improved stress coping and energy levels.** Exercise helps you cope with stress and have more energy.
- **Enhanced mood.** Exercise can improve your mood. If you feel low, take a walk, jump rope, or run up and down the stairs.

GET PHYSICAL

Here are some tips to get you started with exercise and help you ride out cravings:

- **Set aside a regular time for exercise.** Find a time that works with your schedule.
- **Aim for 30 minutes of physical activity most days.** Studies show that exercising for 10 minutes three times a day provides the same benefits as 30 minutes of continuous exercise.
- **Do activities you enjoy.** Walking is one way to get more physical activity. Consider biking, swimming, dancing, or yoga. Even housework or gardening can provide exercise benefits. Playing music while you clean out your closets will help you step up the pace.
- **Build exercise into other activities.** Take the stairs at work instead of the elevator. At the mall, use the stairs instead of the escalator. Wherever you go, park your car farther away and walk to your destination.
- **Plan activities with family, friends, or coworkers that include physical activity.** Consider a hike or a volleyball game.

- **Change your exercise routine or try a new activity occasionally**. This will help prevent boredom.

Incorporating physical activity into your quit plan can effectively manage cravings and reduce withdrawal symptoms. Exercise not only distracts from the urge to smoke but also offers numerous health benefits, including improved mood and reduced appetite. Stay active, try different exercises, and enjoy the journey to a smoke-free life.[1]

[1] Smokefree.gov, "Fight Cravings with Exercise," U.S. Department of Health and Human Services (HHS), July 9, 2016. Available online. URL: https://smokefree.gov/challenges-when-quitting/cravings-triggers/fight-cravings-exercise. Accessed July 11, 2024.

Chapter 34 | **Managing Your Mood after Quitting**

Chapter Contents

Section 34.1 | Smoking, Anxiety, and Mood Changes

It is common to think that smoking calms your nerves and helps with anxiety. However, nicotine can actually cause or worsen anxiety symptoms. Researchers know that nicotine in cigarettes affects your brain and mood. Feelings of fear, nervousness, or panic characterize anxiety. While occasional anxiety is normal, persistent anxiety can lead to sadness, depression, and physical symptoms such as a racing heart or stomach problems.

Some smokers believe that smoking eases anxiety, but this is due to the temporary relief of nicotine withdrawal symptoms. Unless underlying issues are addressed, anxiety is likely to return, perpetuating the cycle.[1]

Smokers are also more likely to experience depression than nonsmokers. Regardless of the cause, effective treatments are available for both depression and smoking.

FIND HELP 24/7

If you or someone you know is in distress or having suicidal thoughts, get help now. Call or text 988 or chat online for 24-hour, free, and confidential support from trained counselors.

MOOD CHANGES AFTER QUITTING

Mood changes are common after quitting smoking. Some people feel increased sadness, irritability, restlessness, or depression. These mood changes may be part of nicotine withdrawal and usually improve within a week or two. If they persist, consult your doctor as it could indicate depression.

Smoking might seem to help with depression temporarily, but it is not a sustainable solution. Here are healthier ways to lift your mood:

- **Exercise.** Being physically active can help. Start small and build up over time. It may be challenging when you are depressed, but the effort will pay off.

[1] Smokefree.gov, "Anxiety and Smoking," U.S. Department of Health and Human Services (HHS), July 9, 2024. Available online. URL: https://smokefree.gov/challenges-when-quitting/cravings-triggers/anxiety-smoking. Accessed July 12, 2024.

- **Structure your day**. Make a plan to stay busy. Get out of the house if you can.
- **Be with other people**. Many people who are depressed isolate themselves. Daily contact with others can improve your mood.
- **Reward yourself**. Do things you enjoy. Even small rewards can help you feel better.

Understanding the connection between smoking, anxiety, and mood changes is essential for those looking to quit. While smoking may offer temporary relief, it ultimately perpetuates anxiety and depression. Healthier coping mechanisms, such as exercise and social interaction, provide more sustainable solutions for improving mood and well-being.[2]

Section 34.2 | Healthy Ways to Cope with Stress after Quitting

MANAGING STRESS AFTER QUITTING SMOKING

Stress is a normal part of life—in moderation, it can help you reach your goals, but too much stress creates more problems. Managing stress is a key part of quitting smoking.

You may have learned to deal with stress by smoking, but there are ways to handle stress without smoking. Here are a few ideas you might find helpful. Some of these tips may take practice, but others you can do right away. Try one or more to learn what works for you.

Relax

Our bodies respond to stress by releasing hormones that increase heart rate and blood pressure. Practicing relaxation techniques

[2] Smokefree.gov, "Smoking and Depression," U.S. Department of Health and Human Services (HHS), June 18, 2024. Available online. URL: https://smokefree.gov/challenges-when-quitting/mood/smoking-depression. Accessed July 12, 2024.

such as the ones below may improve your health and help you handle stress in positive ways.

- **Breathe.** Take a few slow, deep breaths—in through your nose, out through your mouth. You will feel your body start to relax.
- **Locate your stress.** Take a minute to figure out how stress affects your body. Where do you feel tension? Finding ways to reduce that tension will also help your mental stress. A warm bath, a massage, or stretching can help you release built-up tension.
- **Visualize.** Think of a place where you feel safe, comfortable, and relaxed. Picture it as clearly as you can, including imagining what you would feel, hear, and maybe even smell if you were in that relaxing place. Let yourself enjoy being there for a few minutes.

Exercise

Being active releases natural chemicals that improve your mood and reduce stress. Sometimes, a short walk is all it takes to relieve stress—and walking is free!

Talk

You do not have to deal with stress alone. Share your feelings with friends, family, and other important people in your life who can support you in staying smoke-free.

Focus

Life can sometimes be overwhelming. Try not to get caught up in worrying about what is next. Instead, focus on what is happening now, not on what you might have to deal with in the future.

Care

Make an extra effort to take care of yourself. This includes eating a balanced diet, drinking plenty of water, and getting enough sleep.

Decaffeinate

Caffeine can make you feel tense, jittery, and stressed. Cutting back or eliminating caffeine can help reduce stress. Switching to herbal tea or hot water with lemon allows you to enjoy a hot beverage without the caffeine.[1]

DISTRACT YOURSELF WITH KINDNESS

When a craving hits, try distracting yourself by being helpful to a friend, family member, coworker, or complete stranger. Acts like putting your neighbor's newspaper on the porch, making a kind comment to the grocery store checkout person, or holding the door for someone can help you focus on others' needs and manage cravings.

Doing a good deed helps you focus your thoughts outward toward others, taking a step outside your own world for a little while. Performing good deeds can have positive effects on your health, such as reducing stress, which is key to quitting smoking. Being caring toward others helps reduce your own stress and may even help you live longer.

PLANNING ACTS OF KINDNESS

Good deeds are done on purpose. Some good deeds require planning, which helps you pay attention and be mindful of the other person's needs. You might help friends or family members by running errands or helping with childcare. You might also make cookies for someone who did you a favor, clean the house, or cook dinner for an older friend or relative. Planning and executing good deeds can help you understand what makes the other person happy.

VOLUNTEERING AND HELPING STRANGERS

You can also do good deeds for total strangers or volunteer your time, whether it is serving at a soup kitchen, cleaning up litter, or helping elderly people with their groceries.

[1] Smokefree.gov, "Coping with Stress without Smoking," U.S. Department of Health and Human Services (HHS), June 18, 2024. Available online. URL: https://smokefree.gov/challenges-when-quitting/stress/coping-with-stress. Accessed July 12, 2024.

Studies show that one good deed leads to another. If you perform a generous or kind act, you are likely to be happier. The happier you feel, the more likely you are to do another kind act.

Effectively managing stress is crucial for quitting smoking successfully. By practicing relaxation techniques, staying active, and engaging in acts of kindness, you can reduce stress and improve your overall well-being. Remember, quitting smoking is a journey, and managing stress is a key part of that process.[2]

Section 34.3 | **Using Mindfulness to Beat Cravings**

USING MINDFULNESS TO COPE WITH CRAVINGS AND STRESS

Many people who quit smoking find that mindfulness helps them cope with cravings and work through stress and depression. Mindfulness is one more way to help manage withdrawal. Practicing mindfulness can be challenging, and it takes time and practice to reap the benefits. However, incorporating mindfulness into your daily life can help care for your whole self: mind, body, and soul.

Mindfulness involves slowing down to pay attention to what is happening around you at the moment. It means being fully aware of your thoughts, emotions, and physical feelings, as well as what you see, hear, touch, and smell around you. Mindfulness is about letting the present moment be what it is, whether good or bad.

EVERYDAY MINDFULNESS

Practicing mindfulness involves breathing methods and other techniques, such as guided imagery, to relax the body and mind. Guided imagery lets you use all your senses to direct your imagination to

[2] Smokefree.gov, "Do Good to Feel Good," U.S. Department of Health and Human Services (HHS), June 18, 2024. Available online. URL: https://smokefree.gov/challenges-when-quitting/mood/do-good-to-feel-good. Accessed July 12, 2024.

a relaxed, focused state. Mindfulness is a skill you can practice in all areas of your life. Mindfulness can:

- help manage nicotine cravings or feelings of withdrawal when quitting smoking
- reduce stress, anxiety, and depression
- increase positive emotions and enjoyment in daily life
- encourage healthier eating habits
- improve relationships

If you have a busy schedule, it can be hard to slow down and notice the little things. A great way to start practicing mindfulness is to set aside time every day to slow down, pay attention to your breathing, and "reset" yourself. Setting aside even one minute, or several times a day, can have a big effect.

USING MINDFULNESS IN YOUR QUIT JOURNEY

Being mindful can help you get past a craving. If a craving hits, try to:

- **Stop, take a breath, and notice what is happening right now**. How does your body feel? What thoughts are you having? Notice what is happening and take in the experience.
- **Imagine your craving like an ocean wave**. It might feel like it gets bigger and bigger, but eventually, it will become smaller and less intense, just like a wave.
- **Recognize the physical feelings in your body that indicate stress**. Take a moment to step away from what you are doing and notice your breathing.
- **Take a walk outdoors**. Walk slowly and really focus on being present. Notice what you see, hear, and smell.
- **Involve yourself fully in something you enjoy, like a hobby**. You will benefit from keeping your brain busy and having something else to consider instead of the craving.
- **Take a trip to your mind**. Imagine yourself at the beach, in a garden, or in the mountains—anywhere you want. Close your eyes and think about what it would

feel like to be there right now. Enjoy all the little things in this beautiful place. Focusing on something else can help you get through your cravings more easily.

Incorporating mindfulness into your quit journey can effectively manage cravings, reduce stress, and improve overall well-being. By practicing mindfulness techniques and staying present, you can navigate the challenges of quitting smoking and support your journey to a healthier, smoke-free life.[1]

[1] Smokefree.gov, "Practice Mindfulness," U.S. Department of Health and Human Services (HHS), July 9, 2024. Available online. URL: https://smokefree.gov/challenges-when-quitting/stress/practice-mindfulness. Accessed July 12, 2024.

Chapter 35 | **Role of Social Support in Smoking Cessation**

Chapter Contents

Section 35.1 | Navigating Relationships While Quitting Smoking

If you have been smoking for a while, people may know you as a smoker. Deciding to quit does not mean you cannot spend time with your friends and family—even if they still smoke.

Relationships are common reasons why people start or continue to smoke. Maybe you grew up around smokers, and it seemed natural for you to smoke, too. Maybe your partner smokes, and it is a way that you spend time together. The important people in your life can also be key to your success in quitting. You might even be surprised by how much help they can be.

TELL THEM YOU ARE QUITTING

Quitting is hard. It is OK to ask for help. If you let people close to you know you are trying to quit, you can tell them what will help you be successful. Be specific—say exactly what you need from them. Here are some suggestions about what to ask of your friends, family, and coworkers:

- **Be supportive**. Some people may be able to quit on their own, but many need help and support. Ask friends, family, and loved ones to be there for you during this time.
- **Understand your change in mood**. Mood changes are common after quitting smoking. Remind the people around you that this is temporary. You can say, "The longer I go without smoking, the sooner I'll be back to my old self."
- **Offer distractions**. Most people have cravings when they quit smoking. Your friends and family can distract you until the craving passes. Ask them to help you come up with a list of things to do.
- **Celebrate with you**. Ask friends and family to help you celebrate your smoke-free successes, such as throwing away your cigarettes, setting a quit date, and reaching milestones like being smoke-free for three days. Even if you slip or relapse, you can still celebrate all the cigarettes you did not smoke!

- **Quit with you**. Does someone close to you smoke? Quitting can be easier with support, so ask them to quit with you. If they are not ready, ask them not to smoke around you or let you bum a cigarette.

THE POWER OF A PARTNER

Romantic partners can significantly influence whether someone becomes smoke-free. People who receive support from their partners have an easier time quitting. However, some partners may not be supportive or may try to control the smoke-free process. This can lower confidence and make it harder to quit. Every couple is different, but relationships tend to follow four patterns regarding how partners relate to each other about smoking:

- **Involved**. Both partners see smoking as a problem because of health, financial, or other reasons but also know that trying to quit can be hard. Regardless of who is smoking in the relationship, they try to be supportive and understanding.
- **Accommodating**. Both partners see smoking as okay and ensure there are chances to smoke during their everyday activities. This is true even if only one partner smokes.
- **Disengaged**. Both partners see smoking as a choice each partner makes. Even if they both smoke, they often smoke when they are not with each other.
- **Conflictual**. One partner criticizes their partner's smoking habits or their decision to continue or quit smoking. This can cause tension, arguments, and hurt feelings. The stress on the relationship might drive someone to slip up and smoke or even go back to smoking regularly. This may especially be true if smoke breaks have been used in the past to find peace. If this sounds like your relationship, ask for help from people who can be more supportive.

Knowing your partner's beliefs about smoking can help you figure out what support you need to become smoke-free. It can also help you prepare for how your partner might react to your quit attempt. If you think your partner might not understand your quit attempt or will not want you to quit smoking, there are other ways to find the support you need.

Quitting smoking is a challenging journey, but the support of friends, family, and partners can make a significant difference. By clearly communicating your needs, celebrating milestones, and understanding relationship dynamics, you can leverage the power of your support network to achieve a smoke-free life.[1]

Section 35.2 | **Getting Support from Loved Ones to Quit Smoking**

Getting support from your loved ones can make a big difference when you quit. Let them know that you are quitting and tell them what kind of support you need.

TALK TO YOUR FRIENDS AND FAMILY

People who get support from family and friends have an easier time stopping smoking and staying smoke-free. Sources of support for you could be:

- your spouse or significant other
- your children or grandchildren
- other close family members
- friends
- coworkers
- friends who are former smokers
- neighbors
- people in your religious or community groups

[1] Smokefree Women, "Relationships and Quitting," U.S. Department of Health and Human Services (HHS), July 9, 2024. Available online. URL: https://women.smokefree.gov/your-relationships/relationship-quitting. Accessed July 12, 2024.

Let these people know that you will be grateful for their support. Tell them you may not be your usual self for a few days or weeks after you quit.

BE SPECIFIC ABOUT WAYS THEY CAN HELP

Only you know what kind of support will be best for you. Suggest ways your loved ones can help you quit. Here are some "do" and "do not" examples to share with your loved ones.

- Let your loved ones know that these might be ways they can help support you quit:
  - Add to your supply of cigarette substitutes (like chewing gum or healthy foods).
  - Fix your favorite meal or go out to lunch or dinner with you.
  - Help you change routines to avoid temptations to smoke.
  - Help you find ways to keep busy.
  - Celebrate your progress with you.
  - Remind you that things will get easier.
  - Do activities with you that take your mind off smoking, like going to a movie together.
  - Ask how you are doing and let you know they care.
  - Understand if you need to stay away from trigger activities for a while after you quit (such as your weekly card game or bingo).
- Let your loved ones know that these are not ways to help you quit:
  - Nag you about your efforts to quit.
  - Doubt that you can quit or stay smoke-free.
  - Ever offer you a cigarette.
  - Joke about you going back to smoking.
  - Smoke around you, especially when you are unable to easily leave (like in the car or at the dinner table).

HANDLING FRIENDS WHO STILL SMOKE

Dealing with friends who smoke may take extra effort. You may want to point out that just because you are quitting does not mean they have to. The decision to quit is a personal one. You may want to avoid friends who smoke during the first few weeks. You could also offer to drive or have guests over to your home. Your friends may be more likely not to smoke in these situations.

Quitting smoking is a challenging journey, but the support of friends, family, and coworkers can make a significant difference. By clearly communicating your needs and being specific about how they can help, you can create a supportive environment that increases your chances of success.[1]

Section 35.3 | **Building a Smoke-Free Support Network**

CREATING A SUPPORT SYSTEM TO QUIT SMOKING

Surrounding yourself with positive support can make it easier to quit. Find out what you can do to create a network of smoke-free support.

Telling the people in your life about your choice to quit smoking and asking them for help can make a big difference. It is likely that people will be supportive and positive when you tell them you are quitting smoking. But, you may come across others who do not understand or who do not want you to quit. Learn how to deal with the different ways others might react.

KNOW WHO IS ON YOUR SIDE

Surrounding yourself with people who support your choice to quit will increase your chances of staying smoke-free for good. Your family, friends, coworkers, and others can help celebrate successes with you, boost your mood, and distract you from picking up a cigarette. But, what if people you care about do not seem supportive when you tell them you are quitting?

See if these types of people seem familiar, and learn how you can deal with their different reactions.

---

[1] Smokefree.gov, "Friends and Family," U.S. Department of Health and Human Services (HHS), June 18, 2024. Available online. URL: https://60plus.smokefree.gov/support/friends-and-family. Accessed July 12, 2024.

Nonsmokers Who Do Not Get It

People who have never smoked might not understand how difficult it is to quit. They might think that smoking is just a "nasty habit." Or they might say things that can make you feel bad if you slip and have a cigarette or start smoking again. It might be hard, but try to be patient with these people. Here are some more ways to deal with nonsmokers who may not understand:

- **Tell them how to help**. Say exactly what would make you feel supported. You could say, "It would help me a lot if you celebrated my smaller smoke-free victories with me."
- **Be positive**. Thank them for their help and tell them how important their friendship is.
- **State your feelings**. Tell them how you feel when they do something that bothers you. For example, "It makes me feel bad when you talk about a time when I've slipped."

Smokers Who Do Not Want to Quit

Staying friends with smokers who are not ready to quit can be one of the hardest things you do while you quit, especially if you smoked together. Even if they are supportive, it can still be hard to be around them because they might remind you of smoking. This can trigger you to want to smoke. Below are some ways you can stay strong and focused on your goal. Try this:

- **Respect them**. Tell them you respect their choice not to quit and tell them how important your relationship is.
- **Respect yourself**. Talk to them about how important quitting is to you and what you are struggling with, like being around cigarettes and cigarette smoke.
- **Work together on a plan**. Decide on smoke-free zones in shared spaces, and when you are together, ask them to smoke outside. Try to meet in smoke-free places.

Smokers Who Are Not on Your Side

There may be people who are not ready to quit and do not want you to either. They smoke around you and leave their cigarettes out, even when you ask them not to. They may even tell you that they do not think you can quit. This can be discouraging and frustrating, especially if it is someone you want to, or have to, keep a relationship with. You may need a break from this person, but that is not always possible or easy. If you cannot give yourself some distance, try one of these other strategies:

- Remind yourself why you are quitting.
- Join a support group or online community and connect with others who will support you.
- Plan to spend time with this person in places where smoking is prohibited (malls, movie theaters, restaurants), or find smoke-free places you enjoy going solo.
- Lean on the people who are supporting you when the going gets tough.

SOCIAL AND SMOKE-FREE

When you quit smoking, you may need to make a few changes to your regular activities to avoid smoking triggers that could lead to a slip. You might be worried that these changes will affect your social life. Luckily, you can still do things you enjoy while working on quitting:

- **Try to socialize with people who support your decision to quit, especially in the first few weeks after quitting.** This period can be hard and seeing others smoke can be a trigger.
- **You and your friends have plenty of things in common besides smoking.** Remind yourself of those things and incorporate them into your social life.
- **Spend time with people who make you feel good about yourself and want you to succeed.**
- **You may need to avoid certain places while you are quitting—such as bars, certain concert venues, or areas where groups of people are smoking.** Explain to your friends that this change is temporary and that you are not avoiding them but are avoiding situations that might make you slip.

BUDDY UP

If there is someone close to you who smokes, ask them if they want to quit with you. It could be helpful to have someone who understands the challenges of becoming smoke-free. Plus, you will have a built-in support system. If they are not ready to quit, be understanding. Tell them that becoming smoke-free is really important to you. Ask them to help you reach that goal by not smoking around you or letting you bum a cigarette, no matter how badly you may want one.

Quitting smoking is a challenging journey, but the support of friends, family, and coworkers can make a significant difference. By clearly communicating your needs, celebrating milestones, and understanding different reactions, you can leverage the power of your support network to achieve a smoke-free life.[1]

Section 35.4 | Supporting a Loved One in Quitting Smoking

Someone who feels supported is more likely to quit smoking for good. Friends, family members, and significant others can play a big part in helping a person become smoke-free.

Here are some tips that can help you support the person in your life who is quitting smoking. The more you know, the more you can help.

KNOW YOUR RELATIONSHIP STYLE

The way you deal with smoking can affect a person who is trying to quit. It helps to become aware of your relationship style. Your style affects their smoking, their quitting, their health, and yours. Understanding your relationship style can help you understand what both of you may have to change to better deal with their smoking and quitting. For example, you may need to:

- recognize your friend or family member's small successes when quitting

[1] Smokefree Women, "Build Your Smoke-Free Team," U.S. Department of Health and Human Services (HHS), July 9, 2024. Available online. URL: https://women.smokefree.gov/your-relationships/build-your-smokefree-team. Accessed July 12, 2024.

- avoid criticizing them if they slip and have a cigarette
- decide it is time for you to quit smoking, too

START THE CONVERSATION

It can be hard to get someone to talk about quitting smoking. To get a conversation started, look for an opening. Respond positively when someone says:

- "I'm thinking about quitting smoking."
- "My doctor told me that I should quit smoking."
- "I'm pregnant. I should probably quit smoking."
- "My partner is pregnant. I should probably quit smoking for them."
- "My kids are asking me about my cigarettes. I should probably quit smoking for them."

Let them know you think it is great they are considering quitting and that you are ready to help. If you are an ex-smoker, you can draw from your own experience of quitting. Let them know how much better you feel now that you are smoke-free. You might say:

- "I'm so proud of you for trying to quit smoking. I'll help with whatever you need to make it happen."
- "Quitting smoking will be hard, but I know you can do it. Have you set a quit date?"
- "You're not in this alone. Even if it gets tough, I'll be here for you."
- "Quitting smoking is the best thing I ever did! Let me know if you need any tips."

ASK QUESTIONS

Asking open-ended questions can help you understand what a quitting smoker is going through. You might ask:

- "What made you want to start smoking?"
- "What things make you crave a cigarette?"
- "What made you decide to quit smoking?"
- "What things have been stressing you out lately?"
- "What could I do to help make quitting easier for you?"

LISTEN

Quitting smoking is about them—not you. Listen to what they have to say. If you ask a question, be quiet and give them time to answer. Resist the urge to insert your own comments.

DO NOT LECTURE

Lectures, nagging, and scolding will not help your friend or family member quit smoking. It might just put you on their bad side, and they may not come to you for help when they really need it.

Here are some things to avoid when you are trying to help someone quit smoking:

- nagging them about why smoking is bad
- counting the number of cigarettes they smoked
- asking them if they smoked today
- arguing with them about being irritable when they are going through withdrawal
- giving them a hard time if they have a bigger appetite from withdrawal
- getting upset if they slip and smoke a cigarette

BE PATIENT AND POSITIVE

Supporting someone who is trying to quit smoking can be frustrating and exhausting. Focus on staying upbeat. Do not give up on them. Your support is important.

The withdrawal that can come from quitting smoking may make a person moody and irritable. Avoid:

- taking their moods personally
- telling them it was easier to put up with their moods when they were smoking
- suggesting it would be easier for them to just go back to smoking

The cravings a person might face can be hard to deal with. Do not let them lose confidence in quitting. Check in on them and let them know you support them. You might say:

- "I can tell this is hard on you, but I'm proud of you for sticking with it. Let's do something fun to celebrate how far you've come!"

- "It sounds like you're having a rough day. How about I take care of dinner tonight/watch the kids/mow the lawn so you can have some time for yourself? You deserve it."

DO NOT BE TOO HARD ON THEM IF THEY SLIP

Your friend or family member may occasionally slip and smoke a cigarette. They will probably feel guilty, so getting angry with them will not help. Instead, you could:

- tell them you know they can still quit and remind them of all the progress they have made
- help them figure out what triggered the craving that led to the slip
- help them come up with a plan for dealing with the craving if it happens again
- ask if there is anything else you can do to help
- help them keep track of when they slip and be aware of the situations and places that are making quitting difficult

Here are some ways you could respond to a slip:

- "Slips happen. Don't beat yourself up over it! Like anything tough, you learn as you go. Use right now as a time to restart and get back on track."
- "So you slipped. Quitting isn't easy and many people need several tries before they quit for good. You've got this, and I'm here for you."
- "Let's talk about what's triggering you to smoke. That will help you stay on track this time. Just don't smoke that next cigarette!"

CELEBRATE SUCCESSES BIG AND SMALL

Recognize your friend or family member's smoke-free successes and milestones. Staying smoke-free for a day, week, or year are all reasons to celebrate. So are throwing out all the ashtrays in the house, ditching any reminder of cigarettes, and passing on an after-dinner cigarette. Help your friend or family member celebrate by:

- sending flowers or a card
- surprising them with tickets to a concert or show

- giving them a gift card to their favorite store
- making a home-cooked dinner

A compliment can go a long way to recognize the positive changes they have made:

- "The smoke-free life works well for you—you look great!"
- "You make quitting smoking look easy. You should be proud of yourself. I am!"

BE THERE FOR THE LONG HAUL

The challenges of quitting smoking do not end when a person puts down their last cigarette. Cravings can pop up weeks, or even months, later. It is not uncommon for ex-smokers to start smoking again within the first three months of quitting.

Let your friend or family member know you are there for the long haul. Keep celebrating their smoke-free anniversaries and offer distractions to help them deal with cravings. Your ongoing support could be all they need to make this quit attempt their last.[1]

[1] Smokefree.gov, "How to Support Your Quitter," U.S. Department of Health and Human Services (HHS), June 18, 2024. Available online. URL: https://smokefree.gov/help-others-quit/how-to-support-someone-quitting. Accessed July 12, 2024.

Chapter 36 | The Benefits of Calling a Quitline for Smoking Cessation

WHY CALLING A QUITLINE CAN HELP YOU QUIT SMOKING

Quitting smoking is a challenging journey, but you do not have to do it alone. Quitlines offer valuable support, resources, and encouragement that can significantly boost your chances of success. Here are five reasons why calling a quitline can be the key to achieving your goal of becoming smoke-free:

You Can Get Help to Stop Smoking—Free, with No Judgment

If you are thinking about quitting smoking and would like some help, a quitline might be just what you need to succeed. Quitlines provide free coaching over the phone to help you quit smoking.

- When you call 1-800-QUIT-NOW, you can speak confidentially with a highly trained quit coach.
- Quitlines provide many of the services and similar support you get in a stop-smoking class or from your doctor and can be a valuable complement to your doctor's care.
- Quitlines are available throughout the United States.
- Coaching help is available in several languages.

Quit Coaches Help Create a Plan That Can Work for You

Quit coaches are trained to help people who smoke to quit. They understand what you are going through. Many used to smoke themselves. They are all trained to be good listeners and to give callers encouragement, support, and helpful tips. A quit coach will ask questions to find out what type of help interests you. They will also ask about your experience with trying to quit smoking. This information helps them give useful suggestions on the type of program that could work best for you.

Quit Coaches Can Help You Get Quit-Smoking Medicines

Quit coaches can help you connect with quit-smoking medicines through your health insurer or community programs. They may also be able to provide you with these medications for free and send an initial two-week supply to your home.

You Can Get Helpful Tips!

To support your journey to quit, consider the following helpful tips:

- how to deal with cravings and withdrawal
- how to get the right kind of help from your friends and family
- what websites, apps, and texting programs might help you quit
- whether to use quit-smoking medication and how to use it

And the Best Reason of All to Use a Quitline—You Are More Likely to Stay Quit!

Quitlines are proven to increase your chances of quitting successfully and staying quit. A quit coach will work with you to develop a personalized plan for your needs.[1]

COMMON QUESTIONS ABOUT QUITLINES

What If I Prefer to Speak to Someone in a Language Other than English?

Most quitlines can arrange for a translator if you or someone you know who wants to quit speaks a different language.

[1] "Five Reasons Why Calling a Quitline Can Be Key to Your Success," Centers for Disease Control and Prevention (CDC), September 12, 2023. Available online. URL: www.cdc.gov/tobacco/campaign/tips/quit-smoking/quitline/index.html. Accessed July 12, 2024.

Additionally, there are quitlines available for people who speak Spanish, Mandarin, Cantonese, Korean, and Vietnamese:

- **Spanish.** 1-855-DÉJELO-YA (1-855-335-3569).
- **Mandarin and Cantonese.** 1-800-838-8917.
- **Korean.** 1-800-556-5564.
- **Vietnamese.** 1-800-778-8440.

Will They Make Me Feel Bad about Smoking?

Absolutely not! Quitline coaches are hired and trained based on their ability to help you. Many used to smoke themselves, so they understand what you are going through. Your success is theirs, too.

What If I Am Not Sure If I Am Ready to Quit Today?

You do not have to be ready to quit today to call the quitline. Your quit coach can help you explore your worries and doubts about quitting and identify new solutions. Our coaches have helped many people who smoke to successfully quit, and they can help you, too.

What If I Use Other Kinds of Tobacco Products?

Quitline coaches can help you if you are using smokeless tobacco, cigars, hookah, e-cigarettes, or other tobacco products in addition to cigarettes.

What If I Do Not Smoke, but I Want to Help a Friend or Family Member Who Does?

It can be a real challenge to know how best to help a friend or relative who smokes to quit. Maybe they do not want to quit, but their smoking is affecting you. Maybe they smoke inside, and it bothers you. Or maybe you are even worried about their health and the diseases that smoking causes. Maybe they want to quit, and you support them, but you do not know how to help. Quit coaches can help you devise a plan to help them quit.

How Do I Know Using a Quitline Will Help?

Over the past 25 years, many studies have been done on the advantages of quitlines. These studies report that people who call a quitline are more likely to quit and stay quit. Combining counseling and quit-smoking medications such as patches can double or triple your chances of success.

What If I Do Not Like to Talk on the Phone?

There are other ways to quit! Quitlines can help you find out about other quit-smoking services, such as apps and texting programs.

Will They Ask for My Personal Information?

To provide callers with the best care, you will be asked to provide some information about yourself. You may be asked for your contact information during your initial call so that you can be reached for follow-up coaching. In addition, you will be asked about your smoking status and history, as well as past attempts at quitting and what caused you to continue smoking. You may also be asked your age, sex, and race. If you do not feel comfortable answering a question, you can always choose not to answer. All the information you provide will be kept confidential.

Will It Cost Anything?

No. Quitline services are free to callers.

How Can I Learn More about Quitlines?

Call 1-800-QUIT-NOW and ask questions.

Calling a quitline can provide you with the support, resources, and encouragement you need to quit smoking successfully. With free, confidential coaching and personalized plans, quitlines increase your chances of becoming smoke-free and staying that way.[2]

[2] "Top 10 Questions People Ask about Quitlines," Centers for Disease Control and Prevention (CDC), September 12, 2023. Available online. URL: www.cdc.gov/tobacco/campaign/tips/quit-smoking/quitline/top-10-questions-people-ask-about-quitlines.html. Accessed July 12, 2024.

Part 4 | Tobacco Prevention and Control

Chapter 37 | Preventing Initiation of Tobacco Use

TOBACCO USE INITIATION

Because cigarette smoking typically begins during adolescence, tobacco use is often described as a "pediatric disease." Nearly 90 percent of adults in the United States who smoke daily began smoking by age 18, and 98 percent first smoked by age 26. Nicotine is highly addictive; initiation of smoking during adolescence is linked to persistent smoking in adulthood and numerous adverse health effects. Additionally, exposure to nicotine during adolescence may harm normal brain development, which continues until about age 25. Specifically, nicotine exposure during this critical period may impair the development of brain regions involved in attention, learning, and impulse control and may prime the brain for addiction to other drugs.

Understanding trends in youth initiation of tobacco products—including cigarettes, electronic cigarettes, cigars, and smokeless tobacco—helps policymakers allocate prevention resources more effectively. Effective strategies to reduce youth initiation of tobacco use include federal regulation of tobacco products; significant increases in tobacco prices, including excise taxes; smoke-free air laws; restrictions on tobacco advertising and promotion; limiting the availability of tobacco products to youth; mass-media public education campaigns; and full implementation of comprehensive state and community tobacco control programs. On December 20, 2019, legislation was enacted to amend the Federal Food, Drug, and Cosmetic Act, raising the federal minimum age of sale of tobacco products from 18 to 21 years.

MEASURES OF INITIATION

- The percentage of individuals aged 12–25 years who initiated cigarette smoking during the past 12 months.
- The percentage of individuals aged 12–25 years who initiated cigar smoking during the past 12 months.
- The percentage of individuals aged 12–25 years who initiated smokeless tobacco use during the past 12 months.
- The percentage of individuals aged 12–25 years who initiated the use of these tobacco products during the past 12 months.

Note: *Initiation measures include a numerator of the number of adolescents and young adults aged 12–25 years who used the specified tobacco product for the first time in the past 12 months and a denominator of the number of adolescents and young adults aged 12–25 years who did not use the specified tobacco product in their lifetime or who used the specified tobacco product for the first time in the past 12 months. Cigars include premium cigars, little cigars, and cigarillos.*[1]

PREVENTING TOBACCO USE

Increased knowledge of the dangers of tobacco use, attitudes against tobacco use, and support for policies to reduce tobacco use initiation are crucial.

Awareness and Attitudes

- level of awareness of antitobacco media messages
- level of receptivity to antitobacco media messages
- level of support for policies and enforcement of policies to decrease the availability of tobacco to young people
- level of support for creating comprehensive tobacco-free policies in schools and on college and university campuses

[1] "Tobacco Use Initiation," National Cancer Institute (NCI), March 2024. Available online. URL: https://progressreport.cancer.gov/prevention/tobacco/smoking_initiation#jump-links-field-trends-and-most-recent-est. Accessed July 15, 2024.

- proportion of young people who think tobacco companies try to get young people to use tobacco products
- level of perceived harm of traditional, nontraditional, and emerging tobacco products among young people

Restrictions and Enforcement in Educational Institutions

- proportion of schools or colleges/universities implementing 100 percent tobacco-free policies
- proportion of schools or school districts providing tobacco-use prevention that meets the guidelines of Centers for Disease Control and Prevention (CDC)
- proportion of young people participating in tobacco-use prevention activities
- level of reported exposure to school-based tobacco-use prevention that meets CDC guidelines
- perceived compliance with tobacco-free policies in schools and on college/university campuses

Sales and Availability Restrictions

- proportion of jurisdictions with strong policies banning nonsale distribution or free sampling of all tobacco products
- proportion of jurisdictions requiring retail licenses to sell tobacco products
- proportion of jurisdictions controlling the type, location, number, and/or density of tobacco retail outlets
- proportion of jurisdictions banning tobacco vending machine sales
- number and type of enforcement actions issued for violations of restrictions on tobacco product availability
- proportion of jurisdictions regulating sales of other tobacco products
- proportion of jurisdictions with strong public policies for tobacco-free workplaces and other public places
- proportion of states with tobacco control laws preempting stronger local tobacco control and prevention laws

Reducing Industry Influence

- proportion of jurisdictions regulating tobacco advertising
- proportion of jurisdictions regulating consumer-focused tobacco promotions
- proportion of jurisdictions regulating merchant-focused industry promotions
- proportion of jurisdictions with minimum tobacco product price laws
- proportion of jurisdictions with public policies establishing a fee on each tobacco product package to cover government costs
- proportion of jurisdictions limiting tobacco industry sponsorship of public and private events
- number and type of enforcement actions for violations of restrictions on tobacco marketing
- number and type of Master Settlement Agreement violations by tobacco companies

Reducing Susceptibility and Exposure

- proportion of young people thinking tobacco use is cool and helps them fit in
- proportion of young people believing tobacco users have more friends
- proportion of young people overestimating the smoking rate among their peers
- proportion of young people reporting their parents strongly disapprove of tobacco use
- proportion of young people with a favorite tobacco brand
- proportion of young people having never used tobacco but are susceptible to its use
- density of stores selling tobacco
- proportion of young people receiving non-sale distribution or free samples of tobacco products
- proportion of retailers selling tobacco products to youth
- proportion of young people reporting tobacco purchases from retailers

- proportion of youth reporting unsuccessful attempts to purchase tobacco products from retailers
- proportion of youth receiving tobacco products from a social source
- proportion of young people purchasing tobacco products from vending machines
- proportion of young people finding it easy to obtain tobacco products

Reducing Tobacco Industry Influence

- extent and type of retail tobacco advertising
- extent of tobacco industry sponsorship of public and private events
- extent of tobacco advertising in media
- extent of tobacco presence in movies
- extent of pro-tobacco Internet presence
- amount and quality of news media stories about tobacco industry practices and political lobbying
- extent of industry-sponsored tobacco use prevention activities
- amount of tobacco industry contributions to institutions and groups
- amount of tobacco industry campaign contributions to local and state politicians

Increasing Tobacco Prices

- amount of tobacco product taxes and fees
- price paid for tobacco products
- extent and type of consumer-focused industry promotions
- extent and type of merchant-focused industry promotions

REDUCING INITIATION AND PREVALENCE

- average age at which young people first smoked a whole cigarette
- average age at which young people first tried a commercial tobacco product other than cigarettes

- proportion of young people having never tried a tobacco product
- prevalence of tobacco use among young people
- proportion of established young tobacco users
- type and brand preferences of young tobacco users
- proportion of poly-tobacco product use among young people
- level of tobacco use among young people

Addressing tobacco use initiation among youth is critical for reducing the long-term prevalence of smoking and its associated health risks. By implementing comprehensive prevention strategies and increasing awareness of the dangers of tobacco use, we can help prevent the next generation from becoming addicted to nicotine.[2]

[2] "Preventing Initiation of Tobacco Use: Outcome Indicators for Comprehensive Tobacco Control Programs–2014," Centers for Disease Control and Prevention (CDC), 2014. Available online. URL: www.cdc.gov/tobacco/stateand-community/tobacco-control/pdfs/preventing_initiation.pdf. Accessed July 15, 2024.

Chapter 38 | Preventing Tobacco Use among Youth

PREVENTING YOUTH USE OF, AND ACCESS TO, TOBACCO PRODUCTS

The Youth Tobacco Prevention Plan, a focused segment of the Comprehensive Plan, aims to stop youth use of and access to tobacco products, particularly electronic cigarettes (e-cigarettes). Significant regulatory and research efforts related to access, marketing, and education are already underway.

A key component of the Comprehensive Plan for Tobacco and Nicotine Regulation of the U.S. Food and Drug Administration (FDA), the Youth Tobacco Prevention Plan is a series of actions to stop youth use of tobacco products, especially e-cigarettes. This plan focuses on three key areas:

1. Preventing youth access to tobacco products.
2. Curbing marketing of tobacco products aimed at youth.
3. Educating teens and retailers.

MILESTONES

The FDA's enforcement actions and youth education efforts designed to protect kids from the harms of e-cigarettes include:

Access

- conducting more than 1 million retail inspections
- holding individual retail locations and corporate retailers accountable for sales to underage purchasers
- pursuing no-tobacco sales orders to retail locations

- barring retail locations that repeatedly sell to underage purchasers from selling tobacco products for a period of time
- taking action on flavored tobacco products to prevent youth access
- addressing the epidemic of youth e-cigarette use by taking action against 1,300+ retailers and five major manufacturers
- warning retailers for selling e-cigarettes to underage purchasers and taking action against retailers for selling tobacco products to underage purchasers

Marketing

- prioritizing enforcement against products with youth appeal
- finalizing policy prioritizing enforcement against certain unauthorized flavored cartridge-based e-cigarettes that appeal to children
- protecting children from e-liquid dangers by warning companies selling misleadingly labeled and/or advertised e-liquids resembling kid-friendly food products
- requiring manufacturers to provide critical information by sending several information requests related to Juul and other e-cigarette products

Education

- educating youth on the dangers of e-cigarette use through developing a Vaping Prevention and Education Resource Center that provides e-cigarette prevention information in English and Spanish, including lesson plans, activity sheets, and videos, to middle and high school educators
- expanding "The Real Cost" campaign to help ensure teens understand the risks of e-cigarettes
- helping retailers comply with age restrictions by launching a retailer education effort, "This Is Our Watch"

The FDA's Youth Tobacco Prevention Plan is a comprehensive effort aimed at preventing youth access to and use of tobacco products, particularly e-cigarettes. Through rigorous enforcement, targeted marketing restrictions, and widespread education initiatives, the plan strives to protect the health of young people and reduce the prevalence of tobacco use among youth.[1]

[1] "FDA's Youth Tobacco Prevention Plan," U.S. Food and Drug Administration (FDA), January 29, 2024. Available online. URL: www.fda.gov/tobacco-products/youth-and-tobacco/fdas-youth-tobacco-prevention-plan. Accessed July 22, 2024.

Chapter 39 | **Smoke-Free Policies**

Chapter Contents

Section 39.1 | Comprehensive Smoke-Free Policies: Protecting Public Health

OVERVIEW: COMPREHENSIVE SMOKE-FREE POLICIES

Eliminating smoking is the only way to fully protect people who do not smoke from secondhand smoke exposure. Comprehensive smoke-free policies prohibit smoking in all areas of indoor spaces at all times, offering full protection against secondhand smoke. These laws cover workplaces, restaurants, bars, and other public places, helping people quit smoking and preventing youth from starting. Implementing these laws across the United States could prevent many disparities in exposure, illnesses, deaths, and lost productivity.

BENEFITS OF COMPREHENSIVE SMOKE-FREE POLICIES

Reduce Secondhand Smoke Exposure

- Studies have found substantial declines in cotinine, a marker of secondhand smoke, among both hospitality workers and the public following the implementation of smoke-free laws.
- Research shows that smoke-free policies lead to substantial declines in secondhand smoke exposure, with air quality improvements of up to 90 percent in high-risk settings like bars.

Improve Health

- Comprehensive smoke-free laws lead to reductions in coronary events, especially heart attacks.
- These laws are one of the most effective and cost-effective ways to reduce heart disease, the leading cause of death in the United States.
- Smoke-free laws in hospitality venues protect employees and customers, improve indoor air quality, and reduce respiratory symptoms.

Reduce Smoking and Encourage Quitting

- Smoke-free laws can make it easier for people to quit smoking, reducing their risk of disease.
- The Task Force on Community Preventive Services found that smoke-free laws in workplaces increase tobacco use cessation by a median of 6.4 percent and decrease tobacco use prevalence by a median of 3.4 percent.

Prevent Smoking Initiation

- Smoke-free workplaces and communities reduce the likelihood of adolescents and young adults starting to smoke by reducing role models who smoke and decreasing opportunities to smoke.

Increase Adoption of Voluntary Smoke-Free Rules

- Implementing smoke-free laws increases the adoption of voluntary smoke-free rules in homes, which may extend to private vehicles, further protecting nonsmokers, especially children.

HOW SMOKE-FREE POLICIES VARY ACROSS THE UNITED STATES

While exposure to secondhand smoke has declined, not everyone is equally protected by comprehensive smoke-free laws. As of July 1, 2022:

- Only 62.5 percent of the U.S. population is covered by 100 percent smoke-free laws for bars, restaurants, and worksites.
- 28 states, Puerto Rico, the U.S. Virgin Islands, and the District of Columbia have comprehensive smoke-free laws prohibiting smoking in private worksites, restaurants, and bars. Twenty-two states, Puerto Rico, and the U.S. Virgin Islands prohibit smoking in state-regulated gambling venues.
- Twenty-five states, Puerto Rico, and the District of Columbia prohibit the use of e-cigarettes in private worksites, restaurants, and bars. Thirteen of those

jurisdictions also prohibit the use of e-cigarettes in gambling venues.
- Over 1,100 U.S. cities and counties have comprehensive smoke-free laws that prohibit smoking tobacco products in private worksites, restaurants, and bars. Additionally, 1,006 communities prohibit the use of e-cigarettes in smoke-free venues.

Smoke-free laws and policies have high levels of public support and compliance. Studies show they do not negatively affect sales of food and beverage items or employment in the hospitality industry. Although the number of comprehensive smoke-free laws has increased among states over time, variation and unequal protection remain.

WHY SOME POPULATION GROUPS ARE MORE LIKELY TO BE EXPOSED

Uneven protections by smoke-free laws result in disparities in secondhand smoke exposure. Groups more likely to be exposed include non-Hispanic Black people, those living below the federal poverty level, people with less than a college degree, individuals living with someone who smokes inside the home, workers in "blue collar" industries, people living in rental properties, and children aged 3–11.

- Almost two of every five children aged 3–11 years, including more than one in two non-Hispanic Black children, were exposed to secondhand smoke during 2017–2018.
- During 2017–2018, secondhand smoke exposure among non-Hispanic Black people and those living below the poverty level was about twice as high compared to non-Hispanic white people and those living above the poverty level.

Comprehensive smoke-free policies are essential for protecting public health by reducing exposure to secondhand smoke, improving overall health, encouraging smoking cessation, and preventing smoking initiation. While progress has been made, efforts must continue to ensure equal protection for all population groups across the United States.[1]

Section 39.2 | **Protecting Your Family from Secondhand Smoke**

IN YOUR HOME

There is no safe amount of secondhand smoke exposure. The home is the main place where many children and adults breathe in secondhand smoke. To protect yourself and those around you, do not smoke or let anyone smoke in your home or car. Encourage family members to quit smoking.

Smoke from one cigarette can stay in a room for hours. Opening windows and using fans, air conditioners, air purifiers, air fresheners, and ventilation systems does not get rid of secondhand smoke. Smoking in another room, such as a bathroom or bedroom, will not protect children and others from secondhand smoke. Secondhand smoke can still spread through your home via doorways, cracks in walls, electrical lines, ventilation systems, and plumbing. In an apartment building, secondhand smoke can travel between units.

Prohibiting all tobacco use, including electronic cigarettes (e-cigarettes), in the home can set a good example for young people. It can also protect people who do not use e-cigarettes from exposure to e-cigarette emissions, which can contain harmful and potentially harmful substances.

OUTSIDE YOUR HOME

If your child goes to daycare or school, talk to the provider or school officials to ensure they have a tobacco-free policy for all facilities. This type of policy can set a good example for young

[1] "Preventing Exposure to Secondhand Smoke in the Community," Centers for Disease Control and Prevention (CDC), May 15, 2024. Available online. URL: www.cdc.gov/tobacco/secondhand-smoke/community.html. Accessed July 15, 2024.

people and protect children from secondhand smoke and e-cigarette emissions. Examples include:

- tobacco-free school events
- tobacco-free school policies that apply to buildings and grounds and include e-cigarettes

If your state or community has not adopted laws preventing exposure to secondhand smoke in public areas, look for restaurants and other public places that do not allow smoking. "No Smoking" sections in restaurants that separate people who smoke from those who do not smoke do not protect you or your children from secondhand smoke.

Talk to your employer about the benefits of a smoke-free policy in your workplace. Educate others about the benefits of smoke-free laws and policies in public places, workplaces, and housing. If you own or manage a business, adopt a smoke-free policy for employees and customers.

AVOIDING OTHER TOBACCO PRODUCTS

Protecting your loved ones also means not using other types of commercial tobacco products, including e-cigarettes. The aerosol from e-cigarettes is not harmless. It can contain cancer-causing chemicals and heavy metals such as nickel, tin, and lead, among other harmful substances. E-cigarettes are not safe for children, teens, young adults, pregnant adults, or people who do not already use tobacco. The U.S. Food and Drug Administration (FDA) has approved no e-cigarette as a quit-smoking aid. There are proven tools that can help current smokers quit successfully.

QUITTING SMOKING

If you smoke cigarettes, the best decision you can make for your health and your family's health is to quit. Quitting smoking can be hard and may take many tries. The good news is there are more proven tools than ever before to help you quit successfully, including cessation (quit-smoking) medicines and coaching and counseling.[1]

---

[1] "Preventing Exposure to Secondhand Smoke in the Home," Centers for Disease Control and Prevention (CDC), May 15, 2024. Available online. URL: www.cdc.gov/tobacco/secondhand-smoke/home.html. Accessed July 15, 2024.

Chapter 40 | Creating Smoke-Free Environments

Chapter Contents

Section 40.1 | Creating a Smoke-Free Home Environment

WHAT IS SECONDHAND SMOKE?

Secondhand smoke is a combination of smoke from the burning end of a cigarette and the smoke exhaled by a smoker. When someone smokes near you, you are exposed to secondhand smoke. The surgeon general of the United States has concluded:

- There is no safe level of secondhand smoke exposure.
- Cleaning the air and ventilating buildings cannot eliminate secondhand smoke.
- Secondhand smoke causes disease and early death in children and adults who do not smoke.

STATISTICS ON SECONDHAND SMOKE EXPOSURE IN THE UNITED STATES

- Approximately, 58 million nonsmokers (1 in 4) are exposed to secondhand smoke.
- About 2 in 5 children, including 7 in 10 Black children, are exposed to secondhand smoke.
- The home is the main place where children are exposed to secondhand smoke.

HEALTH RISKS OF SECONDHAND SMOKE

For Babies and Children

- sudden infant death syndrome (SIDS)
- lung problems
- ear infections
- asthma attacks

For Adults

- heart disease
- stroke
- lung cancer

DID YOU KNOW?

Secondhand smoke can travel through doorways, cracks in walls, electrical lines, ventilation systems, and plumbing. Only 100 percent smoke-free indoor air fully protects from secondhand smoke exposure. Opening windows, using fans, and relying on heating, air conditioning, and ventilation systems cannot eliminate exposure to secondhand smoke. In fact, these systems can distribute secondhand smoke throughout a building.

KEY TAKEAWAYS

To protect yourself and your family, create a smoke-free home environment. Encourage others to quit smoking and adopt smoke-free policies in your household to ensure the health and well-being of everyone in your home.[1]

Section 40.2 | Comprehensive Smoke-Free Policies in Multiunit Housing Facilities

INTRODUCTION TO SECONDHAND SMOKE EXPOSURE IN MULTIUNIT HOUSING

Secondhand smoke causes premature death and disease in children and nonsmoking adults. Approximately, 58 million individuals in the United States who do not smoke are still exposed to secondhand smoke. The immediate adverse effects of secondhand smoke on the cardiovascular system can cause heart disease, stroke, and lung cancer in nonsmoking adults. Children are particularly vulnerable, facing increased risks of sudden infant death syndrome, acute respiratory infections, middle ear disease, severe asthma, respiratory symptoms, and slowed lung growth. Annually, over

[1] "Going Smoke-Free Matters: In Your Home," Centers for Disease Control and Prevention (CDC), July 27, 2023. Available online. URL: https://data.cdc.gov/api/views/k4xj-uge6/files/ac7da77d-4178-4ab1-951e-d7b58d03c01a?filename=Going+Smokefree+Matters+-+In+Your+Home+Infographic.pdf. Accessed July 22, 2024.

41,000 nonsmoking adults and 400 infants die from exposure to secondhand smoke. Despite significant progress in protecting nonsmokers through state and local laws and employer-imposed smoking restrictions in indoor worksites and public places, many remain exposed in unregulated areas, including their homes. The home is the primary source of secondhand smoke exposure for children, highlighting the need for focused protective measures in residential settings.

RISK AND EXPOSURE IN THE DOMESTIC ENVIRONMENT

There is no risk-free level of secondhand smoke exposure; even brief exposures can negatively affect nonsmokers' health. It is estimated that about 15 million U.S. children aged 3–11 years are exposed to secondhand smoke primarily in their homes. Nearly one in five children in this age group live in homes where smoking occurs indoors, a stark contrast to one in twenty nonsmoking adults. Children in smoking-permitted homes exhibit higher levels of biological markers for secondhand smoke exposure than those in nonsmoking homes. The only effective measure to fully protect nonsmokers from secondhand smoke exposure is the elimination of smoking in indoor spaces.

CHALLENGES OF SMOKE-FREE LIVING IN MULTIUNIT HOUSING

Individuals living in multiunit housing, such as apartments and condominiums, are particularly susceptible to involuntary secondhand smoke exposure. Secondhand smoke can infiltrate throughout a building via various pathways, and exposure levels can vary based on the building's structure, age, and smoking policies. Even with household smoking bans, secondhand smoke from other units and shared areas can enter individual units. Current engineering solutions, including ventilation and air cleaning, are insufficient to fully eliminate the risk of secondhand smoke exposure. Approximately, 80 million residents in the United States live in multiunit housing facilities; among those with smoke-free home rules, an estimated 27.6–28.9 million still face exposure to secondhand smoke from neighboring units or common areas.

LEGISLATIVE EFFORTS AND COMMUNITY RESPONSES

State and local governments have recognized the risks of secondhand smoke infiltration in multiunit housing facilities. Some regions, like Hawaii and Oklahoma, have enacted laws restricting smoking in government-owned multiunit housing facilities, particularly in common areas such as lobbies and hallways. However, exemptions often apply to individual units, undermining the effectiveness of these restrictions. Community surveys in Minnesota and Oregon reflect strong public support for smoke-free living spaces, with a significant majority of residents implementing smoke-free rules in their units and supporting the rights of facility owners to enforce these policies.

FUTURE DIRECTIONS FOR ENHANCING SMOKE-FREE POLICIES

As of March 31, 2024, only 16 states and territories have restrictions on smoking in government or private multiunit housing facilities, predominantly limiting smoking to common areas. Recent educational campaigns have successfully increased the prevalence of smoke-free home rules from 43 percent in 1993 to 83 percent in 2011, demonstrating growing public support for reducing exposure to secondhand smoke. To fully protect residents, 100 percent smoke-free policies in multiunit housing facilities, covering both common areas and individual units, are essential. These policies can be adopted voluntarily by property managers, condominium associations, housing authorities, or through local or state legislation, with local and state governments playing crucial roles in addressing this public health issue.[1]

---

[1] "STATE System Multiunit Housing Fact Sheet," Centers for Disease Control and Prevention (CDC), June 24, 2024. Available online. URL: www.cdc.gov/statesystem/factsheets/multiunithousing/MultiUnitHousing.html#secondhand-smoke-detrimental. Accessed July 22, 2024.

Section 40.3 | Transforming Casinos into Smoke-Free Zones

THE CASE FOR SMOKE-FREE WORKPLACES

Every worker deserves to breathe smoke-free air. However, employees in casinos, bars, and restaurants are disproportionately exposed to toxic secondhand smoke compared to other segments of the U.S. workforce. Notably, 75 percent of regular casino-goers support smoke-free casinos.

THE HEALTH IMPLICATIONS OF SECONDHAND SMOKE

The surgeon general of the United States has clearly stated that there is no risk-free level of secondhand smoke exposure. Efforts such as cleaning the air, creating separate smoking sections, and enhancing building ventilation are insufficient. Heating, air conditioning, and ventilation systems alone cannot eliminate exposure. The only effective measure to prevent secondhand smoke exposure in workplaces is implementing 100 percent smoke-free policies. Health risks associated with secondhand smoke include:

- heart disease
- lung cancer
- respiratory diseases

Each year, exposure to secondhand smoke is responsible for an estimated 41,000 deaths from lung cancer and heart disease among U.S. adults.

BENEFITS OF SMOKE-FREE POLICIES

Smoke-free policies lead to multiple positive outcomes:

- improved air quality
- enhanced public health
- broad public support
- reduced exposure to secondhand smoke
- decreased smoking rates
- high levels of policy compliance

RECOMMENDATIONS FROM HEALTH AUTHORITIES

The National Institute for Occupational Safety and Health (NIOSH) advocates for the establishment of smoke-free areas to protect from both secondhand smoke and emissions from electronic cigarettes, recommending that these policies cover:

- all indoor areas, without exceptions
- areas immediately outside building entrances and air intakes
- all work vehicles

A PERSONAL STORY: THE CONSEQUENCES OF EXPOSURE

The story of Nathan, a Native-American member of the Oglala Sioux tribe, underscores the personal health risks associated with secondhand smoke in workplaces. Despite never smoking himself, Nathan's 11-year tenure at a smoking-permitted casino led to the development of allergies and serious infections that triggered asthma attacks. Eventually, these conditions caused irreversible lung damage known as "bronchiectasis," leading to his death at the age of 54 on October 17, 2013.

The overwhelming evidence and tragic personal stories highlight the urgent need for comprehensive smoke-free workplace policies. Protecting workers from secondhand smoke is not just a health imperative but a fundamental worker right.[1]

Section 40.4 | Smoke-Free Policies in Bars and Restaurants

SMOKE-FREE WORK ENVIRONMENTS

Every worker deserves to breathe smoke-free air. Bar and restaurant workers are more likely to be exposed to secondhand smoke at their job sites than other segments of the U.S. workforce.

[1] "Going Smoke-Free Matters: Casinos," Centers for Disease Control and Prevention (CDC), 2019. Available online. URL: https://data.cdc.gov/api/views/xdg2-nh8n/files/6febdaeb-43ea-415f-9538-5852fbcd89be?filename=Going+Smokefree+Matters+-+Casinos+Infographic_rev2019.pdf. Accessed July 22, 2024.

HEALTH RISKS OF SECONDHAND SMOKE

The surgeon general of the United States concluded that there is no risk-free level of secondhand smoke. Efforts like separating smokers from nonsmokers, cleaning the air, and ventilating buildings cannot eliminate exposure to secondhand smoke. Similarly, heating, air conditioning, and ventilation systems alone cannot eliminate exposure. The only effective measure is 100 percent smoke-free workplace policies.

Secondhand smoke contains 7,000 chemicals, including 70 that cause cancer. Since 1964, 2.5 million nonsmokers in the United States have died from problems caused by secondhand smoke exposure. Exposure in nonsmokers increases the risk of stroke by 20–30 percent and causes an estimated 41,000 deaths from lung cancer and heart disease among adults each year in the United States.

BENEFITS OF SMOKE-FREE POLICIES

Smoke-free policies improve air quality, improve health, receive public support, reduce secondhand smoke exposure, reduce smoking, and result in high levels of compliance.

RECOMMENDATIONS BY THE NATIONAL INSTITUTE FOR OCCUPATIONAL SAFETY AND HEALTH

The National Institute for Occupational Safety and Health (NIOSH) recommends establishing smoke-free areas that protect from secondhand smoke and electronic cigarette emissions. These areas include all indoor areas without exception, all areas immediately outside building entrances and air intakes, and all work vehicles.

Twenty-three states do not yet have comprehensive smoke-free indoor air laws covering all bars, restaurants, and worksites. This underscores the need for broader legislative action to protect public health in these environments.[1]

---

[1] "Going Smoke-Free Matters-Bars and Restaurants," Centers for Disease Control and Prevention (CDC), July 29, 2023. Available online. URL: https://data.cdc.gov/download/e92c-t3mi/application%2Fpdf. Accessed July 24, 2024.

Chapter 41 | Role of Cessation Interventions in Tobacco Control

Chapter Contents

UNDERSTANDING CESSATION INTERVENTIONS

Although a good deal of effective tobacco cessation treatments exist, quitting tobacco is challenging. Most people who smoke make multiple quit attempts before succeeding, and most try to quit independently, resulting in low overall cessation rates.

Population-based cessation interventions aim to facilitate successful quitting by ensuring barrier-free, evidence-based treatments and services are accessible to all who need them. These strategic efforts, which change policies and systems, can dramatically improve health by normalizing quitting and institutionalizing tobacco use screening and treatment in medical care. These interventions include:

- promoting health system changes to integrate tobacco use treatment into routine clinical care
- enhancing insurance coverage for evidence-based cessation treatments and increasing utilization of these covered treatments
- supporting state tobacco quitlines

IMPROVING CESSATION ACCESS

Cessation interventions increase access to evidence-based treatment by ensuring the following:

- Treatment is offered to every person who smokes through accessible and comfortable methods.
- There are no limits or other barriers to treatment.
- People are aware of available treatments.

PROMOTING HEALTH SYSTEMS CHANGE

Since 8 in 10 people who smoke visit a doctor annually, healthcare providers are pivotal in promoting cessation. In 2015, fewer than three in five smokers received advice to quit from a health professional. Providers often face time constraints and may lack training and confidence in delivering cessation interventions. Furthermore, they are not adequately reimbursed for treating tobacco use and may assume patients are resistant to quitting. However, it is crucial for providers to discuss cessation, as people who smoke value doctors' advice, and even brief counseling (under 3 minutes) is effective.

Health systems change strategies involve screening every patient for tobacco use and offering help at every visit. These changes may include revising policies, processes, information technologies, staff training, performance feedback, and quality improvement initiatives to support tobacco use treatment. The goal is to automate screening and treatment, making them routine rather than dependent on provider recall.

Various health-care providers, including those in primary care, emergency medicine, obstetrics and gynecology, dentistry, and behavioral health, can treat tobacco use. Implementing the health systems changes across diverse settings, involving all staff members, enhances effectiveness.

Evidence shows that brief tobacco use treatment during short interactions with providers can help individuals quit permanently and increase the likelihood of future quit attempts. Combining training with reminder systems, like electronic health record (EHR) alerts, enhances provider adherence to screening and follow-up, reducing smoking prevalence and improving patient satisfaction.

HEALTH SYSTEMS CHANGE COMPONENTS

Health systems change is customizable based on each system's characteristics, including financial resources, workflow, staffing, patient population, EHR use, and quality improvement efforts. Components typically include:

- educating health-care leadership, providers, and staff on the importance of treating tobacco use
- integrating tobacco screening and treatment into existing workflows
- referring patients to quitting resources
- creating staff reminders to treat tobacco use
- documenting treatment and sharing results for quality improvement
- reimbursing providers for tobacco use treatment

IMPROVING CESSATION COVERAGE

Comprehensive insurance coverage for cessation treatment boosts the number of people attempting to quit, using evidence-based treatments, and quitting successfully. For example, in Massachusetts, after implementing an evidence-based tobacco cessation benefit for Medicaid enrollees in 2006, smoking prevalence decreased significantly, and hospitalizations for heart-related conditions dropped by nearly half. For every dollar spent on the benefit, Massachusetts saved over three dollars in medical costs for cardiovascular conditions alone.

SUPPORTING STATE QUITLINES

State tobacco quitlines offer free, confidential, evidence-based telephone counseling, significantly increasing the likelihood of successful quitting. They provide individual counseling, practical advice, medication information, and help with quit plans. Services have expanded to include Internet, chat, text messaging, and mobile app options. Quitlines are cost-effective and accessible, operating during evenings and weekends to accommodate diverse schedules.

Despite their effectiveness, state quitlines reach only about 1 percent of smokers annually. Strategies to enhance quitline effectiveness include securing consistent funding and increasing reach among underserved populations.

TAKING A COMPREHENSIVE APPROACH

The described cessation interventions are individually effective and significantly more impactful when implemented together. For instance, comprehensive cessation coverage facilitates health system changes by simplifying providers' roles, and state quitlines can extend treatment effects initiated by health-care providers.[1]

---

[1] "Best Practices User Guide: Cessation in Tobacco Prevention and Control," Centers for Disease Control and Prevention (CDC), 2020. Available online. URL: https://stacks.cdc.gov/view/cdc/125946. Accessed July 22, 2024.

Section 41.2 | Enhancing Tobacco Cessation through Strategic Coverage Expansion

EDUCATING STAKEHOLDERS ON CESSATION COVERAGE

State tobacco control programs are crucial in educating key stakeholders—including private and public health-care systems, health insurers, the state Medicaid program, and employers—about the significance of comprehensive cessation coverage. Educating employers is vital because they can significantly expand cessation coverage by demanding it and, if self-insured, directly providing it.

For cessation insurance coverage to be effective, it must be comprehensive. This includes all evidence-based treatments, such as individual, group, and telephone counseling, along with all seven Food and Drug Administration (FDA)-approved cessation medications (bupropion, varenicline, and five forms of nicotine replacement therapy: patch, gum, lozenge, inhaler, and nasal spray). Comprehensive coverage also involves eliminating or minimizing cost-sharing and other barriers, and proactively promoting the coverage to ensure both smokers and their health-care providers are aware of it, thus enhancing usage.

In January 2011, the Office of Personnel Management (OPM) implemented a cessation benefit for federal employees through the Federal Employees Health Benefits Program, setting a model for comprehensive, evidence-based coverage:

- individual, group, and telephone counseling
- all seven FDA-approved cessation medications, both prescription and over-the-counter (OTC)
- coverage for two quit attempts per year, with four counseling sessions per attempt
- no copays, coinsurance, or deductibles
- no annual or lifetime limits

Once comprehensive cessation coverage is established, state tobacco control programs should work with health-care systems, insurers, employers, and other partners to publicize this coverage to smokers and health-care providers and to monitor its utilization. High utilization is crucial for the effectiveness of a cessation benefit, as even the most comprehensive coverage will have little effect if not widely used or known.

EXPANDING COVERAGE THROUGH STATE AND FEDERAL INITIATIVES

Another strategic direction for state programs is to work with the state Medicaid program to expand Medicaid cessation coverage. State employees, who often comprise a significant portion of the workforce, can benefit from such expanded coverage, which can serve as a model for private employers and health plans. Several states have also mandated that private health insurers provide some level of cessation coverage.

The results of Massachusetts' Medicaid Cessation Benefit implemented in 2006 are noteworthy:

- utilized by about 37 percent of Medicaid recipients who smoked, or more than 70,000 individuals in the first 2½ years
- smoking rate among Medicaid enrollees fell from 38.3 to 28.3 percent
- annual hospital admissions for heart attacks and other acute heart disease diagnoses among users of the benefit fell by 46 and 49 percent, respectively
- return on investment of $3.12 in cost savings from averted hospitalizations for acute cardiovascular events for every dollar spent

The Affordable Care Act (ACA) has provisions that expand private and Medicaid cessation coverage. For example, non-grandfathered private plans are required to cover, without cost-sharing, preventive services that receive an "A" or "B" rating from the United States. Preventive Services Task Force, including tobacco cessation treatments. This requirement also applies to plans in the individual and small group health insurance markets through state Health Insurance Marketplaces.

Furthermore, as of October 2010, the ACA mandates state Medicaid programs to cover cessation counseling for pregnant women and, effective January 2014, to include FDA-approved cessation medications in their coverage for all Medicaid enrollees. States that expand Medicaid eligibility must provide tobacco cessation coverage to newly eligible adults through a benchmark benefit package. State programs are encouraged to ensure these provisions are fully utilized, given the high rates of smoking and its associated costs in the Medicaid population.

ADDRESSING PREMIUMS AND EXPANDING MEDICARE COVERAGE

Another provision of the ACA allows health insurers in the individual and small group markets to charge tobacco users higher premiums, up to a ratio of 1.5 to 1. However, states can reduce this ratio or prohibit the practice entirely. While higher premiums might motivate cessation, they could also lead tobacco users to misrepresent their tobacco use, avoid seeking cessation assistance, or forego health insurance altogether, especially if costs become prohibitive.

Separately, the Centers for Medicare and Medicaid Services have taken steps to expand cessation coverage for Medicare enrollees, now including individual counseling and prescription cessation medications, though not yet offering comprehensive cessation coverage. There are opportunities to promote Medicare cessation benefits to increase their utilization.

SAMPLE STATE ACTIVITIES: EXPANDING INSURANCE COVERAGE OF PROVEN CESSATION TREATMENTS

- Build and maintain relationships with private health insurers, the state Medicaid program, the state employee health plan, and large employers to educate them about comprehensive cessation coverage and its health and economic benefits.
- Ensure that both fee-for-service and managed-care Medicaid plans provide comprehensive cessation coverage.
- Promote and monitor utilization of the state Medicaid cessation benefit.
- Work with state government to ensure that state employees have comprehensive cessation coverage.

- Implement a state mandate requiring private health insurers to provide comprehensive cessation coverage.
- Monitor implementation and effects of the ACA provisions that expand cessation coverage, as well as those that allow health insurers to charge tobacco users higher premiums.[1]

[1] "Cessation Interventions," Centers for Disease Control and Prevention (CDC), March 2, 2014. Available online. URL: https://stacks.cdc.gov/view/cdc/153234. Accessed July 23, 2024.

Chapter 42 | **Media's Role in Tobacco Use**

Chapter Contents

Section 42.1 | Limiting Tobacco Advertising and Promotions

THE INFLUENCE OF TOBACCO ADVERTISING

Tobacco industry advertising and promotions not only depict but also reinforce social norms that support smoking. These tactics contribute to social pressures on young people to start smoking and weaken smokers' resolve to quit. By creating the impression that smoking is more common and socially rewarding than it actually is, and by misleadingly portraying smoking as healthful, these strategies effectively target youths.

STRATEGIES TO LIMIT TOBACCO ADVERTISING AND PROMOTIONS

Various states have implemented strategies to counteract tobacco advertising and promotions:

- Petition and persuade public authorities with regulatory powers to restrict or ban advertising and promotion within their scope of authority, such as on public transportation.
- Encourage property and business owners and managers to voluntarily reject cigarette advertising and tobacco promotion on their premises.
- Urge sponsors of civic, sports, arts, and other events, particularly those appealing to priority populations, to refuse cigarette advertising and promotional sponsorship.
- Persuade media owners and advertising managers to reject cigarette advertising and to publish editorials supporting advertising and promotion bans.
- Provide the media with information on the tobacco industry's advertising strategies, public attitudes supportive of advertising control, and the financial ties of organizations that accept tobacco industry business.

Achieving restrictions on advertising and promotions at the state or local level can be challenging due to First Amendment concerns, federal preemption under the 1965 Federal Cigarette Labeling and

Advertising Act, and the economic interests of the media in preserving advertising revenue. Such economic interests often prevent publishers from highlighting the hazards of tobacco use.

When the ASSIST (American Stop Smoking Intervention Study) program began, it was unclear which policy actions could be legally implemented to restrict tobacco product advertising. Over time, case law on cigarette advertising and promotion has evolved, allowing some actions to be based on precedent, while others required new legal interpretations. For instance, states and communities could prohibit certain forms of advertising and promotion, such as distributing free samples or advertising in municipal venues. However, no state can outright ban cigarette advertising in nationally distributed magazines due to interstate commerce laws.

ASSIST PROGRAM OBJECTIVES

The ASSIST program aimed to achieve four primary outcomes in restricting tobacco advertising and promotions:

1. Enforce permissible state and municipal restrictions, such as bans on advertising on mass transit, in municipal stadiums, and on billboards; restrictions on free samples; and actions under state laws against unfair or deceptive cigarette advertising.
2. Encourage substantial and progressive voluntary actions by media, advertising managers, and event managers to refuse cigarette advertising and promotion.
3. Enhance public and policymaker support for restraints on tobacco advertising and promotion.
4. Increase public awareness of the nature and role of cigarette advertising and promotion.

ASSIST employed several strategies to limit tobacco advertising and promotions, including:

- Convincing property owners to prohibit tobacco advertising on billboards in ballparks and on posters near schools.
- Encouraging sponsors of cultural and sports events to decline tobacco advertising opportunities.

- Engaging in media advocacy to expose factual omissions and distortions in tobacco advertising and coverage.

Although limited in resources for a paid countermarketing campaign, ASSIST staff capitalized on opportunities to gain media coverage that emphasized the health consequences of tobacco use. While such mass media campaigns are known to raise awareness, they typically do not lead to behavior change. The primary goal here was to enhance public awareness.

DEFINITIONS: ACCESS, AVAILABILITY, AND RESTRICTION

In the context of tobacco control policy interventions, the terms access, availability, and restriction are defined as follows:

- **Access**. The ease or difficulty with which individuals can obtain tobacco products. ASSIST aimed to make it more challenging for individuals, especially minors, to purchase tobacco in the community.
- **Availability**. The locations within the community where tobacco products can be purchased or acquired, and how they are displayed in stores. ASSIST sought to limit these locations.
- **Restriction**. Any public or private policy, whether mandatory or voluntary, that reduces the use, possession, promotion, access, or availability of tobacco products in a given location.

The concerted efforts of the ASSIST program illustrate the critical role of both regulatory and voluntary measures in combating tobacco advertising and promotion. By fostering restrictions and encouraging public and private entities to reject tobacco marketing, these strategies can significantly diminish tobacco's social acceptability and influence. Ultimately, these measures are vital for reducing tobacco use and protecting public health, especially among vulnerable populations like youth.[1]

[1] Division of Cancer Control and Population Sciences (DCCPS), "Public and Private Policy Interventions," National Cancer Institute (NCI), 2020. Available online. URL: https://cancercontrol.cancer.gov/sites/default/files/2020-06/m16_6.pdf. Accessed July 23, 2023.

Section 42.2 | The Role of Counter-Marketing in Reducing Tobacco Use

COUNTER-MARKETING IN TOBACCO CONTROL

With the success of programs in states like Arizona, California, Florida, Massachusetts, Minnesota, Mississippi, and Oregon over the past decade, it has become clear that comprehensive tobacco control programs are a powerful tool for reducing tobacco use. Numerous studies have highlighted the crucial role of robust counter-marketing programs within these initiatives. Tobacco counter-marketing employs commercial marketing tactics to diminish the prevalence of tobacco use and aims to neutralize pro-tobacco influences while amplifying pro-health messages across states, regions, or communities.

Counter-marketing efforts are instrumental in increasing smoking cessation, reducing smokeless tobacco use, lowering the likelihood of initiating cigarette smoking, and decreasing nonsmokers' exposure to secondhand tobacco smoke. These messages significantly bolster public support for tobacco control interventions and enhance backing for educational and community initiatives. They are most effective when integrated with local programs across a state.

THE NECESSITY OF COUNTER-MARKETING

Tobacco counter-marketing programs counteract the influential promotional activities of the tobacco industry, which annually spends billions on advertising and promotions. These statistics underline the critical need for tobacco counter-marketing:

- Annual spending on cigarette marketing by the six major U.S. cigarette makers increased by 16.2 percent from 1999 to 2000, rising from $8.24 to $9.57 billion—the highest figure reported to the Federal Trade Commission.
- In 1999, the top five smokeless tobacco companies in the United States spent $170.2 million on advertising and promotions, marking an all-time high.

- In 2000, these companies spent over $949,000 on Internet advertising.
- In 2000, more than 80 percent of young people in the United States were exposed to magazine ads for "youth" brands of cigarettes an average of 17 times per person.
- Approximately one-third of middle school students and one-fourth of high school students in the United States saw tobacco ads online in 2000.

CHARACTERISTICS OF EFFECTIVE COUNTER-MARKETING PROGRAMS

The Best Practices for Comprehensive Tobacco Control Programs (www.cdc.gov/tobacco/stateandcommunity/guides/pdfs/2014/comprehensive.pdf) outlines several elements crucial to effective tobacco control programs, including counter-marketing. Key characteristics of successful counter-marketing campaigns include:

- **Long-term commitment**. Tobacco industry efforts to establish brand identity and normalize tobacco use spanned decades. Similarly, tobacco control must be viewed as a long-term commitment.
- **Integration with tobacco control**. Counter-marketing should complement and be integrated with other elements of tobacco control, such as education, cessation initiatives, and policy campaigns.
- **Cultural competence**. Effective programs must tailor their messages to affect various demographic groups differently affected by tobacco use.
- **Strategic planning**. Managing a counter-marketing program involves strategic decisions about direction, target audiences, creative content, implementation, and evaluation.
- **Ongoing evaluation**. Continuous assessment is vital to adapt and ensure the program meets its goals.
- **Adequate funding**. Intense counter-marketing is necessary to counteract the pervasive pro-tobacco messaging that begins influencing individuals from a young age.

DEMONSTRATED EFFECT OF COUNTER-MARKETING

Successful examples such as the California Tobacco Education Media Campaign and the Florida Pilot Program on Tobacco Control show significant declines in smoking rates and changes in attitudes toward tobacco use among youth. These campaigns integrate media, grassroots marketing, and educational efforts to effectively reduce tobacco consumption and initiation.

Comprehensive, consistent, and culturally tailored counter-marketing is essential for mitigating tobacco's harmful effects. While many aspects of a campaign can be measured and tested, effective counter-marketing also requires an artful touch and strategic finesse.[1]

[1] "Designing and Implementing an Effective Tobacco Counter-Marketing Campaign," Centers for Disease Control and Prevention (CDC), October 2003. Available online. URL: https://stacks.cdc.gov/view/cdc/24176. Accessed July 23, 2024.

Chapter 43 | National and State Tobacco Control Programs

OVERVIEW

Smoking harms nearly every organ of the body, causing many diseases and affecting smokers' health in general. The Office on Smoking and Health (OSH) supports states and communities in implementing comprehensive tobacco control programs. These programs include national and local campaigns and events, links to state and community resources, guidelines, and data compilation.

PROGRAM FORMATION

The OSH established the National and State Tobacco Control Program (NTCP) in 1999. The NTCP fosters coordinated national efforts to reduce tobacco-related diseases and deaths. It provides funding and technical support to state and territorial health departments. The NTCP supports:

- all 50 states
- Washington, DC
- Puerto Rico
- Guam

GOALS OF THE NATIONAL AND STATE TOBACCO CONTROL PROGRAM

The NTCP aims to:

- eliminate exposure to secondhand smoke
- promote smoking cessation among adults and youth

- prevent tobacco initiation among youth and young adults
- advance health equity by identifying and eliminating disparities related to commercial tobacco products

STRATEGIC APPROACHES OF THE NATIONAL AND STATE TOBACCO CONTROL PROGRAM

The NTCP employs several strategies to meet its objectives:

- state and community interventions
- mass-reach health communication interventions
- interventions for tobacco use and dependence treatment
- surveillance and evaluation

SUSTAINING STATE OBJECTIVES

To sustain these efforts, the NTCP focuses on:

- providing strategic consultation to states and territories to sustain their programs
- developing and maintaining partnerships that provide leadership for state and territorial funding continuity
- expanding and providing science around specific best practice components
- developing and providing training for states and territories to support and promote program sustainability[1]

[1] "National and State Tobacco Control Program," Centers for Disease Control and Prevention (CDC), May 15, 2024. Available online. URL: https://www.cdc.gov/tobacco/php/tobacco-control-programs. Accessed July 24, 2024.

Chapter 44 | Commercial Tobacco Use: Addressing Disparities and Seeking Equity

OVERVIEW

Health equity ensures that all individuals have fair and just opportunities to achieve optimal health. This objective necessitates:

- valuing everyone equitably in terms of their health
- confronting systemic issues, unfair practices, and harmful conditions that compromise the health of specific groups
- engaging various groups in culturally sensitive ways to address their unique health challenges

THE TOBACCO INDUSTRY'S EFFECT ON DIVERSE COMMUNITIES

Several factors link commercial tobacco use to increased disease, disability, and mortality among different population groups:

- targeted marketing and advertising by the tobacco industry aimed at specific communities
- use of flavor additives in tobacco products to attract particular demographics
- the exacerbating effects of discrimination, poverty, and other social conditions on tobacco use and health outcomes
- lack of adequate protection against secondhand smoke exposure

- barriers to accessing health care and tobacco cessation treatments

These factors contribute to disparities in tobacco use, secondhand smoke exposure, health issues, and access to treatment, varying by geographic location, employment type, health insurance coverage, and demographic factors such as race, ethnicity, age, sexual orientation, disability status, education level, income, and behavioral health status.

African-American Communities

Commercial tobacco significantly hinders health equity among African-American communities:

- In 2020, 19.4 percent of non-Hispanic Black adults used tobacco products.
- In 2021, 8.2 percent of non-Hispanic Black youth used tobacco, compared to 11.0 percent of non-Hispanic white youth, with notable disparities in cigar use.
- Although African Americans typically start smoking later than whites, they are more likely to die from smoking-related diseases.
- Despite similar rates of smoking, African Americans smoke fewer cigarettes daily.

African Americans face disproportionate health issues and higher mortality rates from smoking-related diseases such as heart disease and diabetes.

Asian, Native Hawaiian, and Pacific Islander Communities

Efforts to combat health disparities in Asian, Native Hawaiian, and Pacific Islander (A/NH/PI) communities must consider the role of commercial tobacco. This group is diverse, encompassing over 50 ethnic and language groups, with varied smoking rates influenced by their countries of origin.

- Native Hawaiian/Pacific Islander adults reported a higher prevalence of cigarette smoking compared to Asian adults in 2019.

- A/NH/PI students showed significant tobacco use, with disparities between various groups.
- Smoking rates differ substantially among Asian populations; for example, Korean adults reported higher rates than Chinese-American adults.

Cigarette smoking increases the risk of cancer and heart disease, leading causes of death in the A/NH/PI community.

Hispanic and Latino Communities

Hispanic/Latino communities encounter unique challenges related to commercial tobacco that obstruct health equity:

- Hispanic adults born in the United States are more likely to smoke than those born abroad.
- Puerto Ricans have higher smoking rates compared to Mexicans and Dominicans in the United States, and Cuban smokers generally consume more cigarettes daily.
- Tobacco use varies among Hispanic youth, with high school students reporting higher usage rates than middle schoolers.

Despite being the nation's second-largest racial/ethnic group, Hispanic communities experience significant disparities in health outcomes related to tobacco use, including higher risks of cancer, heart disease, stroke, and diabetes.

LGBTQ+ Communities

LGBTQ+ individuals face significant health burdens from commercial tobacco:

- In 2020, 16.1 percent of lesbian, gay, or bisexual adults smoked cigarettes—higher than the rate among heterosexual/straight adults.
- Transgender adults have higher rates of e-cigarette use and overall tobacco product use compared to cisgender adults.
- In 2021, tobacco use was notably higher among gay, lesbian, or bisexual middle and high school students compared to their heterosexual peers.

LGBTQ+ adults are at increased risk for cardiovascular diseases and cancers linked to smoking. The LGBTQ+ population also faces higher HIV rates, further complicating health outcomes related to smoking.

Socioeconomic Status and Tobacco

People with low socioeconomic status (SES) experience a disproportionate burden of tobacco-related health issues:

- higher disease incidence and smoking rates among those uninsured or on public insurance
- increased lung cancer risk associated with lower income levels
- greater likelihood of diabetes among smokers from lower SES backgrounds

Substance Use and Smoking

The correlation between smoking and other substance uses is notable:

- Adults who smoke cigarettes report a three times higher prevalence of illicit drug use compared to nonsmokers.
- The rate of binge drinking is nearly double among smokers compared to nonsmokers.
- Among adults newly diagnosed with a substance use disorder, nearly two-thirds are current smokers.
- Over three-quarters of individuals in treatment for illegal drug use and dependency are current smokers.

Geographic Disparities in Tobacco Use

People in the U.S. South and Midwest experience higher rates of tobacco use and related health issues compared to other regions:

- Rural areas report worse health outcomes associated with tobacco use.
- Lung cancer deaths are notably higher in rural areas, largely attributable to smoking.

Reducing tobacco use disparities is vital for advancing health equity and improving outcomes across all populations.[1]

---

[1] "Health Disparities Related to Commercial Tobacco and Advancing Health Equity: An Overview," Centers for Disease Control and Prevention (CDC), May 15, 2024. Available online. URL: www.cdc.gov/tobacco-health-equity/about. Accessed July 23, 2024.

Chapter 45 | Reducing Industry Influence in the Tobacco Retail Environment

Commercial tobacco use, including cigarettes, cigars, smokeless tobacco, and electronic cigarettes (e-cigarettes), remains prevalent in areas where tobacco retailers are concentrated. Communities with a high density of these retailers, often including lower-income populations, youth, and historically marginalized racial and ethnic groups, experience higher rates of tobacco use and greater difficulty in quitting.

Focusing on the local retail environment ensures that strategies to reduce tobacco use are culturally relevant to these communities. Retail strategies are crucial and complement other tobacco control measures to reduce disparities and achieve health equity.

HOW RETAIL STRATEGIES ADVANCE HEALTH EQUITY

- **Reducing access to tobacco products**. Restricting where retailers can sell tobacco products can reduce exposure and differences in retailer density between communities.
- **Reducing exposure to tobacco marketing**. Industry marketing targets specific groups and is more prevalent in certain communities. Reducing exposure to tobacco advertising can denormalize tobacco use and promote cessation.

- **Promoting tobacco cessation.** Equitable retail strategies can help people quit by reducing exposure to advertising, promoting cessation resources, and limiting access to tobacco products. Banning flavors, including menthol, can make it easier for people in high-use communities to quit.

RETAIL STRATEGIES TO REDUCE TOBACCO USE

Product Availability

Reducing the types of tobacco products sold by retailers can have a significant effect.

STRATEGIES

- restricting sales of certain product types, such as flavored tobacco products
- prohibiting the sale of all tobacco products

HEALTH EQUITY EFFECT

- flavor restrictions may reduce youth initiation and menthol-related disparities
- restricting product sales limits the industry's retail presence

Pricing and Promotion

Nontax approaches can reduce the industry's ability to lower product prices.

STRATEGIES

- setting minimum prices for certain pack sizes
- restricting coupon redemption

HEALTH EQUITY EFFECT

- higher prices help prevent youth initiation and motivate people with low incomes to quit
- nontax approaches help reduce disparities and complement taxes

Advertising

Reducing exposure to promotional items and ads based on the time, place, or manner can significantly affect tobacco use.

STRATEGIES

- content-neutral ad restrictions that limit all signage regardless of content
- consulting with a public health attorney before considering any advertising restrictions

HEALTH EQUITY EFFECT

- may reduce tobacco advertising in low-income and minority communities
- decreased exposure to marketing can decrease cravings and impulse purchases

Age of Sale

Raising the minimum age of sale for tobacco products can prevent youth initiation.

STRATEGIES

- restricting sales to people over the age of 21 to support enforcement of the federal Tobacco 21 law
- prohibiting Internet sales of tobacco products

HEALTH EQUITY EFFECT

- may reduce underage sales in low-income and minority neighborhoods
- raising the minimum age may prevent young people from purchasing for themselves or others

Retail Licensure

Implementing, evaluating, and enforcing retail strategies through licensing or zoning policies, including lowering retailer density, is essential for effective tobacco control.

STRATEGIES

- **Capping.** Limiting the number of retailers to balance their distribution across neighborhoods.
- **De-clustering.** Restricting retailers from operating near each other.
- **Proximity.** Restricting where retailers can be located, such as away from schools or at adult-only retailers.

HEALTH EQUITY EFFECT

- may reduce retailer concentration in low-income and minority communities
- decreasing retail density may reduce exposure to marketing that targets certain populations
- capping the number of retailers, especially around schools, can more equitably reduce density

OVERCOMING POTENTIAL CHALLENGES

Industry opposition and preemption are common challenges communities face when implementing retail strategies. Dispelling myths spread by the tobacco industry and understanding preemption can help overcome these obstacles.

Dispel Myths about Retail Strategies

The tobacco industry and convenience store associations often oppose retail restrictions on economic grounds. However, the evidence does not support these claims. Retail strategies can effectively reduce tobacco-related disparities and promote health equity, with little to no effect on retailers' profits. Retail policies will unlikely cause small retailers to go out of business, as customers who would otherwise buy tobacco will spend money on other goods. Nontobacco products, such as snacks and beverages, are more profitable than tobacco products.

The industry has also tried to encourage opposition by aligning itself with the communities it targets, claiming that tobacco control strategies are discriminatory. They sometimes use front groups to oppose strategies, a tactic known as "astroturfing."

Programs can play an important role in educating about industry influence in the retail environment. Participating in public hearings, holding press conferences, or giving presentations can be effective ways to:

- counter myths and share facts, especially with retailers
- raise awareness about industry tactics and their effect on tobacco-related disparities
- share how retail strategies can improve community health and reduce disparities

Implementing retail strategies to reduce commercial tobacco use is essential for promoting health equity and reducing disparities in affected communities. By addressing product availability, pricing, promotion, and advertising, these strategies can effectively diminish tobacco use and support cessation efforts. Overcoming industry opposition and dispelling myths will ensure the success of these initiatives, leading to healthier communities.[1]

[1] "Tobacco Where You Live: Retail Strategies to Promote Health Equity" Centers for Disease Control and Prevention (CDC), 2022. Available online. URL: https://stacks.cdc.gov/view/cdc/125973/cdc_125973_DS1.pdf. Accessed July 24, 2024.

Chapter 46 | Challenges and Strategies in Global Tobacco Control

Tobacco use remains a leading global cause of preventable premature death, including deaths from cancer. Globally, there are over 1.1 billion tobacco smokers aged 15 and older, imposing more than US$1 trillion annually in health-care costs and lost productivity. Despite the availability of effective, evidence-based interventions to reduce tobacco use and related morbidity and mortality, these measures are underutilized.

EVIDENCE AND CHALLENGES IN LOW- AND MIDDLE-INCOME COUNTRIES

The research presents new findings from low- and middle-income countries (LMICs), highlighting the unique challenges of implementing tobacco control measures in these regions. It examines global tobacco control efforts following the adoption (2003) and enactment (2005) of the World Health Organization Framework Convention on Tobacco Control (WHO FCTC). The discussion also covers infrastructure issues from privatization to trade liberalization and evolving trends in tobacco use and the tobacco product market.

HEALTH AND ECONOMIC BURDEN

The global health and economic burden of tobacco use is substantial, increasingly borne by LMICs, where around 80 percent of the world's smokers reside. Annually, tobacco use causes approximately

6 million deaths, a number projected to rise to about 8 million by 2030, with over 80 percent of these deaths occurring in LMICs.

ECONOMIC RATIONALE FOR GOVERNMENT INTERVENTION

Market failures in tobacco products provide an economic rationale for government intervention. These failures include the public's imperfect knowledge about the health and economic consequences of tobacco use, asymmetric information availability, and the effect of tobacco use on nonusers, such as exposure to secondhand smoke and public health-care costs for tobacco-related diseases.

POLICY AND PROGRAMMATIC INTERVENTIONS

Effective policy and programmatic interventions are available but underutilized. The WHO FCTC offers an evidence-based framework for government action to mitigate tobacco use. Interventions to reduce tobacco demand are highly cost-effective, including significant increases in tobacco taxes and prices, comprehensive bans on tobacco industry marketing, prominent pictorial health warning labels, smoke-free policies, and population-wide tobacco cessation programs. In 2013–2014, global tobacco excise taxes generated nearly US$269 billion in government revenues, yet less than US$1 billion was spent on tobacco control.

Controlling the illicit trade in tobacco products, now governed by its own international treaty, is crucial for reducing tobacco use and its health and economic consequences.

MARKET POWER AND ECONOMIC EFFECTS

The market power of tobacco companies has increased, posing new challenges for tobacco control efforts. Over the last 25 years, the global tobacco market has become more concentrated, with five companies dominating 85 percent of the global cigarette market. Tobacco control does not harm economies; the number of jobs dependent on tobacco has been falling in most countries, primarily due to technological innovation and globalization. Tobacco control measures generally have modest effects on tobacco-related employment and do not result in net job losses.

REDUCING HEALTH DISPARITIES

Tobacco control reduces the disproportionate burden tobacco use imposes on the poor, who are increasingly the main users of tobacco. Tobacco use contributes to poverty, which itself is a risk factor for poor health. Tobacco control interventions can reduce tobacco use and help alleviate health disparities.

CONTINUING EFFORTS AND SURVEILLANCE

Significant progress has been made in controlling the global tobacco epidemic, particularly in LMICs, but continued efforts are needed to maintain or accelerate this progress. This includes ongoing research and surveillance, implementation of evidence-based tobacco control strategies, and vigilant monitoring of the tobacco industry's efforts to promote tobacco use and undermine control measures.[1]

[1] Division of Cancer Control and Population Sciences (DCCPS), "The Economics of Tobacco and Tobacco Control," National Cancer Institute (NCI), January 15, 2024. Available online. URL: https://cancercontrol.cancer.gov/sites/default/files/2020-08/monograph-flyer.pdf. Accessed July 24, 2024.

Chapter 47 | The Evolving Landscape of Tobacco Use and Control

Tobacco use remains the leading cause of preventable disease, disability, and death in the United States unless the prevalence of tobacco use, especially of combustible products, is reduced more rapidly than the current trajectory. Such reductions require coordinated efforts to prevent initiation among young people and to create an environment that supports cessation among current users. Significant progress has been made, but more can be done—and with enhanced expediency. To end the tobacco use epidemic, evidence-based strategies must be fully implemented and sustained with sufficient intensity and duration. Without this, nearly half a million Americans will continue to die each year from smoking-related diseases and exposure to secondhand smoke, and millions will continue to live with serious smoking-related diseases, costing society hundreds of billions of dollars in smoking-attributable health-care expenditures and lost productivity.

CHALLENGES TO ACHIEVING A TOBACCO-FREE SOCIETY

Marked disparities exist in tobacco product use, and some subpopulations face a considerably higher burden of tobacco-associated morbidity and mortality. Tobacco use remains higher among males, middle-aged adults, American Indians/Alaska Natives, persons with lower levels of education, those living below the poverty level, residents of the Midwest and South, individuals without health insurance or insured through Medicaid, sexual and gender minorities, persons with disabilities, and those with behavioral health conditions. Additionally, disparities in cessation persist across population groups, with lower prevalence of key indicators of cessation—such as quit attempts, advice to quit from a health professional, and access to cessation therapies—among some vulnerable subgroups. For instance, uninsured smokers and Hispanic smokers are less likely to receive advice to quit from a health professional, and they, along with gay/lesbian/bisexual smokers, are less likely to use cessation counseling and/or medication as part of a quit attempt. To eliminate these disparities, tobacco control programs and policies, including barrier-free access to cessation treatments, must be implemented equitably.

ADDRESSING INDUSTRY INFLUENCE AND MARKETING TACTICS

Disparities in tobacco use and cessation are compounded by the tobacco industry's aggressive marketing and promotion of addictive and lethal products, aimed at retaining current users and recruiting new consumers, including youth and young adults. Such marketing and promotional activities have significantly contributed to disparities in cigarette smoking and cessation. The tobacco industry's deceptive nature has been underscored by reports highlighting that the tobacco epidemic has been sustained by aggressive industry strategies that deliberately mislead the public about the risks of smoking.

THE CHANGING TOBACCO PRODUCT LANDSCAPE

The tobacco product landscape continues to evolve, now including various combustible, noncombustible, and electronic products. For example, heated tobacco products have reentered the U.S. market. More research is needed to understand the long-term health effects of these products, as preliminary data suggest certain heated products have lower levels of harmful ingredients than conventional cigarettes. However, concerns remain about the sustained dual use of heated and conventional products, youth initiation, and the limited number of independent studies assessing these products' potential health risks.

The diversification of tobacco products could affect cessation rates among adults and progress in reducing use among youth.

Electronic cigarette (e-cigarette) brands have emerged, with many now owned by cigarette manufacturers. The increasing availability and use of novel tobacco products, especially e-cigarettes, raise questions about their effect on efforts to eliminate tobacco-related disease and death. While e-cigarettes might help some adult smokers quit, the potential risks, particularly the increase in youth using e-cigarettes and becoming addicted to nicotine, could offset any benefits.

PUBLIC HEALTH CONSIDERATIONS AND E-CIGARETTES

Electronic cigarettes could potentially help adult smokers if they completely switch from conventional cigarettes to e-cigarettes. However, any potential population-level benefits would need to outweigh the risks related to increased youth initiation. E-cigarette use among U.S. high school students has surged, driven by products such as Juul, which deliver nicotine in the form of nicotine salts, allowing for higher nicotine levels with less irritation. This introduces additional risks since nicotine is highly addictive and can harm adolescent brain development.

For e-cigarettes to be effective harm-reduction tools, smokers must completely quit conventional cigarettes and eventually also quit using e-cigarettes. While evidence on e-cigarettes and smoking cessation is growing, the majority of e-cigarette users also smoke conventional cigarettes, which does not significantly reduce individual risk. Studies on e-cigarettes' efficacy for smoking cessation are emerging, but findings may not be generalizable to all settings due to varying levels of nicotine dependence, reasons for e-cigarette use, and differing regulatory environments.

THE NEED FOR COMPREHENSIVE RESEARCH AND EVIDENCE-BASED RECOMMENDATIONS

Comprehensive and evidence-based research is needed to understand e-cigarettes' long-term health effects and their influence on cessation. Given the evolving landscape of e-cigarettes, including the introduction of nicotine salts, research on different types of products and usage frequencies is essential. Public health recommendations must be based on robust evidence that considers the potential negative effects of promoting e-cigarettes for cessation, especially regarding youth initiation.

To achieve a net public health gain, any benefits of e-cigarette use among adult smokers must outweigh the risks of increased initiation among youth. A balanced approach, considering both potential benefits and risks, is crucial in developing effective tobacco control strategies.[1]

[1] "Smoking Cessation: A Report of the Surgeon General," U.S. Department of Health and Human Services (HHS), 2020. Available online. URL: www.hhs.gov/sites/default/files/2020-cessation-sgr-full-report.pdf. Accessed July 22, 2024.

Part 5 | Additional Help and Information

Chapter 48 | Glossary of Terms Related to Tobacco Use and Smoking Cessation

absorption: The process of taking in. For a person or an animal, absorption is the process of a substance getting into the body through the eyes, skin, stomach, intestines, or lungs.

ACE inhibitor: A drug that is used to lower blood pressure. An ACE inhibitor is a type of antihypertensive agent. Also called "angiotensin-converting enzyme inhibitor."

acquired immunodeficiency syndrome (AIDS): A disease caused by the human immunodeficiency virus (HIV). People with AIDS are at an increased risk for developing certain cancers and for infections that usually occur only in individuals with a weak immune system.

addiction: A chronic, relapsing disease characterized by compulsive drug seeking and use despite serious adverse consequences, and by long-lasting changes in the brain.

adverse effect: An unexpected medical problem that happens during treatment with a drug or other therapy. Adverse effects may be mild, moderate, or severe, and may be caused by something other than the drug or therapy being given. Also called "adverse event."

alcohol: A chemical substance found in drinks such as beer, wine, and liquor. It is also found in some medicines, mouthwashes, household products, and essential oils (scented liquid taken from certain plants). It is made by a chemical process called "fermentation" that uses sugars and yeast.

antibiotic: A drug used to treat infections caused by bacteria and other microorganisms.

This glossary contains terms excerpted from documents produced by several sources deemed reliable.

anxiety: Feelings of fear, dread, and uneasiness that may occur as a reaction to stress. A person with anxiety may sweat, feel restless and tense, and have a rapid heartbeat.

arthritis: A general term for conditions that cause inflammation (swelling) of the joints and surrounding tissues. Some forms of arthritis may occur simultaneously with osteoporosis and Paget disease.

assessment: The process of gathering evidence and documentation of a student's learning.

asthma: A chronic disease in which the bronchial airways in the lungs become narrowed and swollen, making it difficult to breathe. Symptoms include wheezing, coughing, tightness in the chest, shortness of breath, and rapid breathing.

backbone: The bones, muscles, tendons, and other tissues that reach from the base of the skull to the tailbone. The backbone encloses the spinal cord and the fluid surrounding the spinal cord. Also called "spinal column," "spine," and "vertebral column."

bacteria: A large group of single-cell microorganisms. Some cause infections and disease in animals and humans.

blood: A tissue with red blood cells (RBCs), white blood cells (WBCs), platelets, and other substances suspended in fluid called "plasma." Blood takes oxygen and nutrients to the tissues, and carries away wastes.

bone: A living, growing tissue made mostly of collagen.

breast cancer: Cancer that forms in tissues of the breast. The most common type of breast cancer is ductal carcinoma, which begins in the lining of the milk ducts (thin tubes that carry milk from the lobules of the breast to the nipple).

calcium: A mineral that is an essential nutrient for bone health. It is also needed for the heart, muscles, and nerves to function properly and for blood to clot.

calorie: A measurement of the energy content of food. The body needs calories as to perform its functions, such as breathing, circulating the blood, and physical activity. When a person is sick, their body may need extra calories to fight fever or other problems.

cancer: A term for diseases in which abnormal cells divide without control and can invade nearby tissues. Cancer cells can also spread to other parts of the body through the blood and lymph systems.

cannabis: The dried leaves and flowering tops of the Cannabis sativa or Cannabis indica plant. Cannabis contains active chemicals called "cannabinoids" that cause drug-like effects all through the body, including the central nervous system and the immune system.

carcinogen: A substance that can cause cancer.

chewing tobacco: A type of shredded or twisted smokeless tobacco that the user keeps in his or her mouth, between the cheek and gum.

chromosome: A chromosome is an organized package of deoxyribonucleic acid (DNA) found in the nucleus of the cell. Different organisms have different numbers of chromosomes. Humans have 23 pairs of chromosomes—22 pairs of numbered chromosomes, called "autosomes," and one pair of sex chromosomes, X and Y.

chronic disease: A disease that has one or more of the following characteristics: is permanent; leaves residual disability; is caused by nonreversible pathological alternation; requires special training of the patient for rehabilitation; or may be expected to require a long period of supervision, observation, or care.

chronic obstructive pulmonary disease (COPD): A type of lung disease marked by permanent damage to tissues in the lungs, making it hard to breathe. COPD includes chronic bronchitis, in which the bronchi (large air passages) are inflamed and scarred, and emphysema, in which the alveoli (tiny air sacs) are damaged. It develops over many years and is usually caused by cigarette smoking.

chronic pain: Pain that can range from mild to severe, and persists or progresses over a long period of time.

cigar: A tube of tobacco that is thicker than a cigarette, wrapped in tobacco leaf, lit, and smoked. Cigars include regular cigars, cigarillos, and little filtered cigars.

cigarette: A tube-shaped tobacco product that is made of finely cut, cured tobacco leaves wrapped in thin paper. It may also have other ingredients, including substances to add different flavors.

computed tomography (CT): A procedure for taking x-ray images from many different angles and then assembling them into a cross-section of the body. This technique is generally used to visualize bone.

constipation: A decrease in frequency of stools or bowel movements with hardening of the stool. Some forms of osteogenesis imperfecta are associated with increased risk for constipation caused by increased perspiration, growth impairment, pelvic malformation, and diminished physical activity.

coronary heart disease: A disease in which there is a narrowing or blockage of the coronary arteries (blood vessels that carry blood and oxygen to the heart). Coronary heart disease is usually caused by atherosclerosis (a buildup of fatty material and plaque inside the coronary arteries).

diabetes: A disease in which the body does not produce or properly use insulin. Insulin is a hormone that is needed to convert sugar, starches, and other food into energy. Having diabetes may increase osteoporosis risk.

diet: What a person eats and drinks. Any type of eating plan.

dip: Dipping tobacco (so called because users dip their fingers into the package to pinch a portion to insert into the mouth) is moist ground tobacco placed between the lower lip or cheek and the gums; it is not used nasally.

dissolvables: Dissolvables are finely ground tobacco pressed into shapes such as tablets, orbs, sticks, or strips and slowly dissolve in the mouth.

dopamine: A brain chemical, classified as a neurotransmitter, found in regions that regulate movement, emotion, motivation, and pleasure.

e-cigarette: A device that has the shape of a cigarette, cigar, or pen and does not contain tobacco. It uses a battery and contains a solution of nicotine, flavorings, and other chemicals, some of which may be harmful.

enzyme: A protein that speeds up chemical reactions in the body.

estrogen: A type of hormone made by the body that helps develop and maintain female sex characteristics and the growth of long bones.

exercise: A type of physical activity that involves planned, structured, and repetitive bodily movement done to maintain or improve one or more components of physical fitness.

fracture: Broken bone. People with osteoporosis, osteogenesis imperfecta, and Paget disease are at greater risk for bone fracture.

head and neck cancer: Cancer that arises in the head or neck region (in the nasal cavity, sinuses, lips, mouth, salivary glands, throat, or larynx [voice box]).

hookah: Hookahs are water pipes that are used to smoke specially made tobacco that comes in different flavors, such as apple, mint, cherry, chocolate, coconut, licorice, cappuccino, and watermelon. Also called "water pipes."

immune system: A complex system of cellular and molecular components having the primary function of distinguishing self from not self and defense against foreign organisms or substances.

inflammatory bowel disease (IBD): Diseases, including ulcerative colitis (UC) and Crohn disease, that cause swelling in the intestine and/or digestive tract, which may result in diarrhea, abdominal pain, fever, and weight loss. People with IBD are at an increased risk for osteoporosis.

inhalation: The act of breathing. A hazardous substance can enter the body this way.

lesion: An area of abnormal tissue. A lesion may be benign (not cancer) or malignant (cancer).

lung cancer: Cancer that forms in tissues of the lung, usually in the cells lining air passages. The two main types are small cell lung cancer and non-small cell lung cancer. These types are diagnosed based on how the cells look under a microscope.

lupus: A chronic inflammatory disease that occurs when the body's immune system attacks its own tissues and organs. Also, called "systemic lupus erythematosus (SLE)." Inflammation caused by lupus can affect many different body systems including joints, skin, kidneys, blood cells, heart, and lungs. People with lupus are at increased risk for osteoporosis.

magnetic resonance imaging (MRI): A noninvasive procedure that uses magnetic fields and radio waves to produce three-dimensional computerized images of areas inside the body.

marijuana: The dried leaves and flowering tops of the Cannabis sativa or Cannabis indica plant. Marijuana contains active chemicals called "cannabinoids" that cause drug-like effects all through the body, including the central nervous system and the immune system.

menopause: The cessation of menstruation in women. Bone health in women often deteriorates after menopause due to a decrease in the female hormone estrogen.

metabolism: The chemical changes that take place in a cell or an organism. These changes make energy and the materials cells and organisms need to grow, reproduce, and stay healthy. Metabolism also helps get rid of toxic substances.

neurotransmitter: A chemical produced by neurons that carry messages from one nerve cell to another.

nicotine: Chemical in tobacco that causes and maintains the powerful addicting effects of tobacco products.

nutrition: The taking in and use of food and other nourishing material by the body. Nutrition is a 3-part process. First, food or drink is consumed. Second, the body breaks down the food or drink into nutrients.

oral cancer: Cancer that forms in tissues of the oral cavity (the mouth) or the oropharynx (the part of the throat at the back of the mouth).

organ: A part of the body that performs a specific function. For example, the heart is an organ.

osteoporosis: Literally means "porous bone." This disease is characterized by too little bone formation, excessive bone loss, or a combination of both, leading to bone fragility and an increased risk of fractures of the hip, spine and wrist.

over-the-counter (OTC): Refers to a medicine that can be bought without a prescription (doctor's order). Examples include analgesics (pain relievers), such as aspirin and acetaminophen. Also called "nonprescription" and "OTC."

overweight: Overweight refers to an excessive amount of body weight that includes muscle, bone, fat, and water. A person who has a body mass index (BMI) of 25 to 29.9 is considered overweight.

periodontitis: A chronic infection that affects the gums and the bones that support the teeth. Bacteria and the body's own immune system break down the bone and connective tissue that hold teeth in place. Teeth may eventually become loose, fall out, or have to be removed.

physical activity: Any bodily movement that is produced by the contraction of skeletal muscle and that substantially increases energy expenditure.

pipe: A tube with a small bowl at one end that is filled with tobacco, lit, and smoked.

portion size: The amount of a food served or eaten in one occasion. A portion is not a standard amount.

pregnancy: The condition between conception (fertilization of an egg by a sperm) and birth, during which the fertilized egg develops in the uterus. In humans, pregnancy lasts about 288 days.

prevention: Actions that reduce exposure or other risks, keep people from getting sick, or keep disease from getting worse.

prognosis: The likely outcome or course of a disease; the chance of recovery or recurrence.

prostate cancer: A disease in which abnormal tumor cells develop in the prostate gland. Men who receive hormone deprivation therapy for prostate cancer have an increased risk of developing osteoporosis and broken bones.

protein: A molecule made up of amino acids. Proteins are needed for the body to function properly. They are the basis of body structures, such as skin and hair, and of other substances such as enzymes, cytokines, and antibodies.

radiation: Energy moving in the form of particles or waves. Familiar radiations are heat, light, radio, and microwaves.

rheumatoid arthritis (RA): An inflammatory disease that causes pain, swelling, stiffness, and loss of function in the joints. It occurs when the immune system, which normally defends the body from invading organisms, attacks the membrane lining the joints. Studies have found an increased risk of bone loss and fracture in individuals with RA.

saliva: The watery fluid in the mouth made by the salivary glands. Saliva moistens food to help digestion and it helps protect the mouth against infections.

secondhand smoke: Smoke that comes from the burning of a tobacco product and smoke that is exhaled by smokers. Inhaling secondhand smoke is called "involuntary" or "passive smoking." Also called "environmental tobacco smoke" and "ETS."

serum: The liquid part of blood that remains after clotting proteins and blood cells are removed.

smokeless tobacco: A type of tobacco that is not smoked or burned. It may be used as chewing tobacco or moist snuff, or inhaled through the nose as dry snuff. Smokeless tobacco contains nicotine and many harmful, cancer-causing chemicals. Using it can lead to nicotine addiction and can cause cancers of the mouth, esophagus, and pancreas. It may also cause heart disease, gum disease, and other health problems.

smoking cessation: To quit smoking. Smoking cessation lowers the risk of cancer and other serious health problems. Counseling, behavior therapy, medicines, and nicotine-containing products, such as nicotine patches, gum, lozenges, inhalers, and nasal sprays, may be used to help a person quit smoking.

snuff: Finely ground smokeless tobacco usually sold in round cans. Can be placed between the cheek and gum or may be sniffed.

snus: Moist snuff packaged in ready-to-use pouches that resemble small tea bags Pouch is placed between cheek or teeth and gums; does not require spitting.

sodium: A mineral and an essential nutrient needed by the human body in relatively small amounts (provided that substantial sweating does not occur).

tobacco: A plant with leaves that have high levels of the addictive chemical nicotine. After harvesting, tobacco leaves are cured, aged, and processed in various ways. The resulting products may be smoked (in cigarettes, cigars, and pipes), applied to the gums (as dipping and chewing tobacco), or inhaled (as snuff).

toxic: Causing temporary or permanent effects detrimental to the functioning of a body organ or group of organs.

virus: In medicine, a very simple microorganism that infects cells and may cause disease. Because viruses can multiply only inside infected cells, they are not considered to be alive.

withdrawal: Symptoms that occur after chronic use of a drug is reduced abruptly or stopped.

x-ray: A type of radiation used in the diagnosis and treatment of cancer and other diseases. In low doses, X-rays are used to diagnose diseases by making pictures of the inside of the body.

Chapter 49 | Smoking Cessation: Hotlines, Helplines, and Internet Resources

NATIONWIDE SMOKING CESSATION HOTLINES AND HELPLINES

American Cancer Society (ACS)
Toll-Free: 800-ACS-2345
(800-227-2345)
Toll-Free TDD/TTY:
866-228-4327
Website: www.cancer.org

American Lung Association
Toll-Free: 800-LUNGUSA
(800-586-4872)
Website: www.lung.org

National Cancer Institute's Smoking Quitline
Toll-Free: 877-44U-QUIT
(877-448-7848)
Website: www.cancer.gov

STATE-BY-STATE HELP FOR SMOKING CESSATION

Alaska
Toll-Free: 800-QUIT-NOW
(800-784-8669)

Arizona
Toll-Free: 800-556-6222
Website: www.ashline.org

Resources here were compiled from several sources deemed reliable; all contact information was verified and updated in August 2024.

California
Toll-Free: 800-300-8086
Spanish: 800-600-8191
Vietnamese: 800-778-8440
Mandarin and Cantonese:
800-838-8917
Korean: 800-556-5564
Website: kickitca.org

Colorado
Toll-Free: 800-QUIT-NOW
(800-784-8669)
Website: www.coquitline.org

Connecticut
Toll-Free: 800-QUIT-NOW
(800-784-8669)
Website: portal.ct.gov

Delaware
Toll-Free: 866-409-1858
Website: dhss.delaware.gov/dhss/dph/dpc/quitline.html

Florida
Toll-Free: 877-U-CAN-NOW
(877-822-6669)
Website: sumter.floridahealth.gov

Georgia
Toll-Free: 877-270-STOP (877-270-7867; in-state calls only)
Toll-Free TDD/TTY: 877-777-6534
Website: dph.georgia.gov/readytoquit

Illinois
Toll-Free: 800-QUIT-YES
(800-784-8937)
Website: quityes.org

Iowa
Toll-Free: 800-QUIT-NOW
(800-784-8669)
Website: iowa.quitlogix.org

Maine
Toll-Free: 800-207-1230

Maryland
Toll-Free: 800-QUIT-NOW
(800-784-8669)
Website: https://quitnow.net/maryland?qnclient=maryland

Massachusetts
Toll-Free: 800-QUIT-NOW
(800-784-8669)
Spanish and Portuguese:
800-8-Déjalo (800-833-5256)
TDD/TTY: 888-229-2182
Website: makesmokinghistory.org/quit-now/what-is-the-helpline

Michigan
Toll-Free: 800-QUIT-NOW
(800-784-8669)
Website: www.michigan.gov/healthymichigan/people/smoking/links

Mississippi
Toll-Free: 800-QUIT-NOW
(800-784-8669)
Website: https://quitnow.net/mve/quitnow

Montana
Toll-Free: 800-QUIT-NOW
(800-784-8669)
Website: benefits.mt.gov/Live-Life-Well/Wellness-Programs/Tobacco-Cessation

Nevada
Toll-Free: 800-QUIT-NOW (800-784-8669)
Website: dpbh.nv.gov/Programs/TPC/dta/Tobacco_Cessation/Tobacco_Cessation

New Jersey
Toll-Free: 866-NJSTOPS (866-657-8677)
Website: njquitline.org

New Mexico
Toll-Free: 800-QUIT-NOW (800-784-8669)
TTY: 877-777-6534
Website: www.nupacnm.com/quitting

New York
Toll-Free: 866-NY-QUITS (866-697-8487)
Website: www.nysmokefree.com

Ohio
Toll-Free: 800-QUIT-NOW (800-784-8669)
Website: odh.ohio.gov/wps/portal/gov/odh/know-our-programs/tobacco-use-prevention-and-cessation/cessation

Oklahoma
Toll-Free: 800-QUIT-NOW (800-784-8669)
Spanish: 855-DÉJELO-YA
TDD/TTY: 877-777-6534
Website: okhelpline.com

Oregon
Toll-Free: 800-QUIT-NOW (800-784-8669)
Website: smokefreeoregon.com/resource/i-want-to-quit

Pennsylvania
Toll-Free: 800-QUIT-NOW (800-784-8669)
Website: www.health.pa.gov/topics/programs/tobacco/Pages/Quitline.aspx

Rhode Island
Toll-Free: 800-QUIT-NOW (800-784-8669
Website: www.health.ri.gov/healthrisks/tobacco/about/quitsmoking

South Dakota
Toll-Free: 866-SD-QUITS (866-737-8487)
Website: www.sdquitline.com

Virginia
Toll-Free: 800-QUIT-NOW (800-784-8669)
Spanish: 855-DEJELO-YA (855-335-3569)
TTY: 877-777-6534
Website: www.vdh.virginia.gov/tobacco-free-living/quit-now-virginia

West Virginia
Toll-Free: 800-QUIT-NOW (800-784-8669)
Website: dhhr.wv.gov/wvdtp/quitline/Pages/default.aspx

Wisconsin
Toll-Free: 800-QUIT-NOW (800-784-8669)
Website: quitline.wisc.edu

ADDITIONAL ONLINE RESOURCES

Clinical Guidelines for Prescribing Pharmacotherapy for Smoking Cessation
Website: www.ahrq.gov/professionals/clinicians-providers/guidelines-recommendations/tobacco/prescrib.html

Committed Quitters
Website: www.quit.com

Guía para Dejar de Fumar
Website: www.cdc.gov/tobacco/campaign/tips/spanish/dejar-fumar/index.html

It's Not Too Late to Quit Smoking
Website: www.cancer.org/cancer/latest-news/never-too-late-to-quit-smoking.html

Kick Butts Day
Website: kickbuttsday.org

Nicotine Anonymous
Website: www.nicotine-anonymous.org

Pathways to Freedom
Website: pathways.thinkport.org

QuitNet
Website: quitnet.com

Smokefree.gov
Website: www.smokefree.gov

Tackling Tobacco
Website: journal.paho.org/en/special-issues/tackling-tobacco-control-beyond-health-comprehensive-approach

Chapter 50 | Resources for Information about Smoking Concerns

GOVERNMENT ORGANIZATIONS

Agency for Healthcare Research and Quality (AHRQ)
5600 Fishers Ln.
7th Fl.
Rockville, MD 20857
Phone: 301-427-1364
Website: www.ahrq.gov

Center for Substance Abuse Prevention (CSAP)
5600 Fishers Ln.
Rockville, MD 20857
Phone: 240-276-2420
Website: www.samhsa.gov

Centers for Disease Control and Prevention (CDC)
1600 Clifton Rd.
Atlanta, GA 30329-4027
Toll-Free: 800-CDC-INFO
(800-232-4636)
Toll-Free TTY: 888-232-6348
Website: www.cdc.gov

Federal Trade Commission (FTC)
600 Pennsylvania Ave., N.W.
Washington, DC 20580
Phone: 202-326-2222
Website: www.ftc.gov

National Cancer Institute (NCI)
9609 Medical Center Dr.
Bethesda, MD 20892-9760
Toll-Free: 800-4-CANCER
(800-422-6237)
Phone: 301-435-3848
Website: www.cancer.gov
Email: NCIinfo@nih.gov

Resources in this chapter were compiled from several sources deemed reliable; all contact information was verified and updated in August 2024.

National Institute on Drug Abuse (NIDA)
16071 Industrial Dr.
Dock 11
Gaithersburg, MD 20892
Phone: 301-443-6441
Website: www.nida.nih.gov

NIH News in Health
9000 Rockville Pike
Bldg. 31, Rm. 5B52
Bethesda, MD 20892
Phone: 301-451-8224
Website: newsinhealth.nih.gov
Email: nihnewsinhealth@od.nih.gov

Office of the Surgeon General (OSG)
200 Independence Ave., S.W.
Humphrey Bldg.
Ste. 701H
Washington, DC 20201
Website: www.surgeongeneral.gov

U.S. Department of Agriculture (USDA)
1400 Independence Ave., S.W.
Washington, DC 20250
Phone: 202-720-7025
Website: www.usda.gov

U.S. Department of Health and Human Services (HHS)
200 Independence Ave., S.W.
Washington, D.C. 20201
Toll-Free: 877-696-6775
Website: www.hhs.gov

U.S. Food and Drug Administration (FDA)
10903 New Hampshire Ave.
Silver Spring, MD 20993-0002
Toll-Free: 888-INFO-FDA (888-463-6332)
Website: www.fda.gov

U.S. National Library of Medicine (NLM)
8600 Rockville Pike
Bethesda, MD 20894
Toll-Free: 888-FIND-NLM (888-346-3656)
Phone: 301-594-5983
Website: www.nlm.nih.gov
Email: NLMCommunications@nih.gov

PRIVATE ORGANIZATIONS

American Cancer Society (ACS)
270 Peachtree St.
N.W., Ste. 1300
Atlanta, GA 30303
Toll-Free: 800-ACS-2345
(800-227-2345)
Website: www.cancer.org

The American College of Obstetricians and Gynecologists (ACOG)
409 12th St., S.W.
Washington, DC 20024-2188
Toll-Free: 800-673-8444
Phone: 202-638-5577
Website: www.acog.org
Email: resources@acog.org

American Heart Association (AHA)
7272 Greenville Ave.
Dallas, TX 75231
Toll-Free: 800-AHA-USA1
(800-242-8721)
Website: www.heart.org

American Lung Association (ALA)
55 W. Wacker Dr.
Ste. 1150
Chicago, IL 60601
Toll-Free: 800-LUNGUSA
(800-586-4872)
Website: www.lung.org
Email: info@lung.org

American Medical Association (AMA)
330 N. Wabash Ave.
Ste. 39300
Chicago, IL 60611-5885
Toll-Free: 800-621-8335
Website: www.ama-assn.org
Email: msc@ama-assn.org

Association of State and Territorial Health Officials (ASTHO)
2231 Crystal Dr.
Ste. 450
Arlington, VA 22202
Phone: 202-371-9090
Fax: 571-527-3189
Website: www.astho.org

Cancer Research Foundation of America (CRFA)
333 John Carlyle St., Ste. 635
Alexandria, VA 22314
Toll-Free: 800-227-2732
Website: www.preventcancer.org
Email: PCF@preventcancer.org

National Center for Tobacco-Free Kids
1400 I St., N.W.
Ste. 1200
Washington, DC 20005
Phone: 202-296-5469
Fax: 202-296-5427
Website: www.tobaccofreekids.org
Email: info@tobaccofreekids.org

National Families in Action (NFIA)
P.O. Box 133136
Atlanta, GA 30333-3136
Phone: 404-248-9676
Website: www.nationalfamilies.org

National Federation of State High School Associations
P.O. Box 690
Indianapolis, IN 46206
Phone: 317-972-6900
Website: www.nfhs.org

National Governors Association (NGA)
444 N. Capitol
Ste. 267
Washington, DC 20001-1512
Phone: 202-624-5300
Website: www.nga.org
Email: info@nga.org

Robert Wood Johnson Foundation (RWJF)
50 College Rd. E.
Princeton, NJ 08540-6614
Toll-Free: 877-843-7953
Phone: 609-627-6000
Website: www.rwjf.org

SmokeFree.net
Website: www.smokefree.net
Email: info@smokefree.net

Truth Initiative
900 G St., N.W.
4th Fl.
Washington, DC 20001
Phone: 202-454-5555
Website: truthinitiative.org

INDEX

INDEX

Page numbers followed by "n" refer to citation information; by "t" indicate tables; and by "f" indicate figures.

A

B

C

Index

D

E

F

G

H

I

K

L

M

N

O

P

Q

T